"When we bring a mindful [...], we enter a path of authentic heali[...]de to transforming our relationshi[...]our spirit."

—**Tara Brach,** author of *Radical Acceptance* and *Radical Compassion*

"A beautiful and poetic guide to awakening our senses, inhabiting our bodies, and opening our hearts to the richness of life. I highly recommend!"

—**Shauna Shapiro, PhD,** author of *Good Morning, I Love You*

"*Savor Every Bite* hits all the right notes. Its goal is to teach readers not only how to recover from dysregulated eating but how to enjoy life more. Rossy does this by laying out a path to whole-body engagement using thoughts, feelings, and senses. Guiding the reader through a five-step process and simple, targeted practice exercises, this empowering book makes change seem less frightening and more doable."

—**Karen R. Koenig, LCSW, MEd,** award-winning
international author of eight books on eating, weight,
and body image (https://www.karenrkoenig.com)

"This book takes a compassionate look at our lifetime relationship to food and eating. We find ways to identify the authentic need behind our cravings. Rossy gives us doable practices to bring a mindful pause to our food choices and a mindful attentiveness to our bodies, too. I was also impressed by how we can find the Dharma on a table or in a mirror."

—**David Richo, PhD,** author of *Triggers: How We Can
Stop Reacting and Start Healing*

"I love these bite-sized chapters and embodied practices. You can read all you like about mindfulness, but it won't take root until you feel it in your body. Lynn Rossy's *Savor Every Bite* helps you do just that with compassion, the benefits of her personal experience, and the backing of scientific data!"

—**Jenna Hollenstein, MS, RDN,** nutrition therapist,
meditation teacher, and author of *Eat to Love*

Savor
Every
BITE

Mindful Ways to
Eat, Love Your Body, and Live with Joy

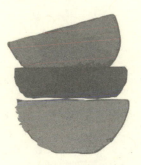

Lynn Rossy, PhD

New Harbinger Publications, Inc.

*To all beings who live in bodies that they
need to feed and care for.*

*May these practices guide you in the art of
eating, moving, and living with joy.*

Contents

Introduction

When we were born, we were delivered without operating instructions. And somewhere along the way, the most instinctual acts we perform—such as eating and moving our bodies—have become quite complicated and confusing. This little book does not provide a set of rules for you to follow; rather, you'll find short, powerful practices in how to become present with your own internal wisdom and knowing heart. Inside of you is the teacher for almost all you need to know. Your body is the expert. Your heart is the guide. You can relearn how to listen to their soft and gentle voices pointing you toward nourishment and restoration.

Modern society, conditioned largely by the diet culture, has taken us away from this inner knowing and replaced it with its ever-changing advice about how to eat, how to look, and how to succeed in being the "perfect self." Modern society functions on a belief system that promotes being thin as the only healthy size, endorses weight loss as the road to happiness, dictates foods you should and should not eat, and harshly judges people who don't match a particular image of beauty. But the diet culture's motto could well be "seek but do not find," as there is always something more or different you need to do in order to be okay. It is the mind-set of "not enough," no matter what you do or how you look.

The journey you take by reading and practicing with this book will help you end the struggle with food, your body, your emotions, and your entire life, as you learn to acknowledge, understand, and the play of emotions that run through your life—from understanding their nature to using your body, mind, and heart to hold them with compassion and tenderness. While food is often used in response to difficult emotions, mindfulness teachings and practices can provide more satisfying responses to the difficulties that will inevitably arise in your life. Step Three: Surrender Limiting Thoughts outlines ten common thoughts that create obstacles to mindful eating and barriers to having a loving relationship with food and your body. Understanding that these thoughts, and subsequent beliefs, are only habits that can be changed liberates you from acting on them and offers you an opportunity to use a beginner's mind when you approach the table, your body, and your life. Step Four: Smile and Create Your Own Happiness helps you realize the power you have to cultivate positive emotions, maintain happier states of mind, and have gratitude for the abundance that is all around you. By cultivating happiness in ways besides eating, you exponentially widen your repertoire for pleasure and find lasting contentment that doesn't disappear when the food is gone. Step Five: Savor Every Moment teaches you the art of appreciating a deep connection to food, movement, nature, health, family, friends and more. Savoring can happen in each moment of intentional presence. Learn to have your cake and eat it too, while you dance to the music of your life!

How to Read This Book

Reading and, most importantly, *practicing* with the exercises in this book from beginning to end will give you a holistic program for

Slow Down and Explore Your Senses

In an age of acceleration, nothing can be more exhilarating than going slow.

—Pico Iyer

If you feel a lot of urgency to fix the way you eat, fix your body, or fix your life, you probably have the feeling of going around in circles without getting anywhere. The truth is there is nothing to fix, but much to explore with curiosity and kindness. By first slowing down, you are placing yourself in the perfect position to hear the answers from within that tell you what you need to know about the food you eat, what your body wants and needs, and the truth of who you are.

Slowing down and exploring your senses as you eat is only the beginning. As you learn to luxuriate in the moments you have with food and your body, your entire life naturally becomes suffused with the beauty of mindful attention and love. Slowing down helps you notice more, and what you notice can teach you volumes about the most important aspects of life. The answers are already waiting for you; all you need to do is slow down to listen.

anxieties—to be smaller, smarter, taller, thinner, quicker, younger, and better-looking. The idea of perfection is both unattainable and, frankly, unnecessary, but the conditioning that tells us we aren't enough is extremely strong and pervasive. Slowing down and experiencing the moments of our lives is ultimately more satisfying than striving for an illusion of success or perfection.

At one point in my life, I went fast because slowing down meant facing things about my life that I didn't want to look at. I thought if I ran fast enough I wouldn't have to face the pain and disappointment of divorce. Of course, that strategy didn't work well at all, and I ultimately ended up in the hospital to recover from drug addiction. Slowing down requires that we be willing to face our lives and our conditioning unflinchingly. You might not like the first image you see in the mirror, but as you begin to spend time with yourself, with kind attention, the truly amazing person you are can begin to shine back at you.

To live fully in the present moment and wake up to our senses requires that we put on the brakes a little. You can't experience the ride when the landscape is whizzing by and you're missing the essential information you need to create the life you want. Slowing down helps you to notice how you are feeling, what you are thinking, and the sensations in your body (such as hunger and fullness) as well as the sights, smells, and sounds around you. These messages are guideposts to your life.

In my yoga classes, I often have people take a deep breath in as they bring their arms overhead. Then I ask them to lower their arms very slowly on a long out-breath. This turns out to be so hard for some people that I repeat it a few times until everyone can

More Savoring Practices: Liberally practice slowing down in other activities. Slow down when you eat (you'll enjoy it more and probably notice you eat less!). Slow down when you're driving and actually drive the speed limit, if traffic allows (I'm still working on this one!). Slow down when you're talking (people might understand you better). Think of other things you do too fast. Slow down, even a little, and notice the difference in how you feel.

worries, doubts, and fears. It's no surprise, then, that research indicates living in the past or the future is associated with increased symptoms of depression and anxiety.

The reason that waking up is hard to do, according to neuroscientists, is that "mind wandering" is the brain's default mode of operation. We are particularly adept at letting our minds stray away from the present; this sets us apart from other species. Reflecting on the past helps us to guide our behavior and consciously plan and prepare for the future. Unfortunately, most of our journeys away from the present take us on a random stroll through a plethora of negative thoughts, and we become significantly less happy as a result.

Another interesting aspect of the research is that even being present for something unpleasant is less difficult emotionally than being lost in thought. In fact, mind wandering itself was found to be generally the cause, and not merely the consequence, of unhappiness. Being present for what's unpleasant in our lives might sound like bad advice, but it actually helps us (much more on this in step two). Denying or repressing your emotions won't get rid of them, and you will probably find yourself engaging in behaviors, like eating when you're not hungry, to mask what's going on inside.

The good news is that you can train yourself to live more in the present. Our next Savoring Practice is A Taste of Mindfulness—a short exercise that can serve as an essential tool for getting back in touch with yourself. Use it throughout the day, particularly before you eat, when you're stressed, and for a sacred pause at any time. Just a little taste of mindfulness is sometimes all you need to tap into

When you know what your body feels like, what feelings are present, and what thoughts are going through your mind, you've dropped out of automatic pilot.

For a moment, sit and breathe and experience being alive. When your mind gets lost in a story, bring your attention back to the passing sensations of body and breath. It doesn't matter how many times your mind wanders. The important thing is to notice, without judgment, and bring your attention back. Each time your mind wanders and you notice is a moment of waking up to the present. Sit, breath, and simply be. When you're ready, open your eyes.

After you open your eyes, reflect whether there was anything of importance or interest that you noticed during the exercise. You might have discovered something that your body, heart, or mind needs as you move into the rest of your day. Repeat the exercise daily for best results!

To support your practice, use the Taste of Mindfulness recorded meditation at http://www.LynnRossy.com/multimedia.

body for waking up so that you can have another day to live. This is where I personally experience a slight smile spreading across my face.

Taking a few moments to be grateful for your body can have miraculous effects. When you get out of bed, take that attitude of gratitude into the rest of your life. Be aware of the sensations of warmth from the sun, of taste as you eat your breakfast and drink your coffee or tea, of love as you greet your family and friends, of meaning as you participate in whatever work you do. None of this would be available to you if you didn't have your precious body. Through your body you experience the gift of life.

I'm not suggesting that you deny the inevitable challenges your body will experience, but I am suggesting that you also remember the score of things that are going well, often without your doing anything to make them happen. Your body virtually operates on its own. The lymphatic system helps the body fight infection, the endocrine system regulates your hormones, the circulatory system moves blood, nutrients, oxygen, carbon dioxide, and hormones around the body, and so on. You help keep your body operating at its best with sleep, food, water, and movement, but it's pretty much on cruise control. Taking a moment to pause and consider these life-giving performances can help us slow down and recognize the powerful vessel that we inhabit.

In working with people and their bodies for over twenty years, I have realized, time and again, that changing how you view your body can generate an improved view of your entire life. One of my students, Ginny, said, "I have learned to be grateful for everything about my body and what it does for me. My body has given birth

4. Breathe with Me

When you find yourself rushing around, feeling stressed out or overwhelmed, you might be tempted to feel better by engaging in behaviors that bring about more harm than healing. For instance, in all of the surveys I've conducted, stress is the number one emotional reason that people reach for food. However, engaging in activities like eating, shopping, drinking, binge-watching TV, checking Facebook, venting, and overworking when you're overwhelmed or emotional provide only temporary relief, and then you're still left with the stress you started with.

The breath is one of the most powerful tools that you have at your fingertips—or your nostrils, to be more exact. Life can get so busy and overwhelming at times that your breath may become so shallow that you are barely getting enough oxygen to your brain and your body to function well. At this point you will be activating the fight-or-flight response. Fighting or fleeing, which is what the body is prepared to do when you become stressed, is rarely a helpful response to the challenges you face in modern life. Can you imagine fighting your coworker or fleeing down the halls of your office when you get overwhelmed?

The fight-or-flight response is a great mechanism when we need to fight for our lives or run from a lion, tiger, or bear, but it has limited use in our day-to-day activities. You can feel the benefits of this hard-wired response when swerving out of the way of a car that gets too close or pulling your child out of danger. Yet it also activates every time you feel a little stress from reading email, listening

While I've been writing this chapter, I have been breathing in lots of fresh air from the open windows. I feel ready to tackle the world!

Savoring Practice

Sit comfortably and bring your hands to your belly. Notice whether your belly is moving in response to your breath. Although you don't actually breathe into your belly, when you let your belly expand you allow your diaphragm to drop down and bring more air into your lungs. Breathe in and out through your nostrils. Let your belly be soft and expand as you breathe in, and pull your belly in as you breathe out. Now, begin to slowly count to four as you breathe in and then breathe out for a count of four—matching the lengths of your inhales and exhales. As you continue, your breath might get deeper and you can increase the number. Continue to breath in this way and notice how you feel. This is called an equal breath (or *sama vritti pranayama* in yoga) and should feel relaxing and calming. Just remember not to strive or push too hard. You don't want to cause yourself more stress by trying to breathe too deeply or too long.

bodies' needs. While this way of eating might seem inaccessible, particularly if you have been dieting for a long time, it is possible to relearn the body cues guiding you to eat this way.

We show love for our belly when we feed it when it is hungry and not so often when it's not. Giving your belly more food than it actually needs to satisfy your body's nutritional needs has consequences. Besides the obvious effect overeating has of uncomfortably expanding your belly, the extra food pushes against other organs in your body and creates discomfort as well as fatigue and drowsiness. Overeating requires your organs to work harder to break down the extra food and may result in heartburn and gas. Overeating regularly can lead to GERD (gastroesophageal reflux disease). And overeating can make it hard for you to sleep through the night, because your circadian rhythms are altered.

When people are stressed or experiencing a difficult emotion, they are particularly vulnerable to increasing the amount they eat, and, according to research, the food they often reach for is high in sugar or fat, or both, even when they are not hungry. Stopping to check in with your belly helps you understand whether you are experiencing signs of stress or hunger. We often experience signs of stress in the belly, and these can be similar to the signs of hunger. However, stress registers as an upset stomach or like someone punched you in the gut, whereas hunger is experienced more as emptiness, gurgling, rumbling, or growling.

You may automatically reach for food at times of stress, but some of these foods (caffeine, artificial and refined sugars, highly processed foods, alcohol, soda) can actually increase your anxiety. In fact, the next time you find yourself eating (or drinking) to relieve

More Savoring Practices: The body wants food when it is physically hungry. When it is stressed, it benefits from activities like stretching, deep breaths, a walk around the block, a conversation with a friend, a little music, dancing, or even a quick nap. Think about other things you can do when you're stressed. This list might be different when you're at work versus at home versus in social situations. Make three lists that reflect these settings. For example, at work, I can walk around the building or up and down the stairs; at home, I can put on music and dance or sit a moment to breathe; and in social situations, I can walk away from the food table, put a napkin over my plate, or engage in conversation.

I fell in love with the practice of "sit down and just eat" at a meditation retreat. One of my biggest pleasures of going on a meditation or yoga retreat is that there is plenty of time to eat—at least an hour. I have the pleasure of eating alone (because often the meals are consumed in silence), and the meals are vegetarian, organic, locally sourced, and prepared by loving hands. There is hardly anything more luxurious than having meals ready and waiting for you and all of the time in the world to eat. Taste seems to explode from the food, as each bite is filled with wonder and nourishment.

The BASICS of Mindful Eating provide a guideline for you to practice "sit down and just eat." The BASICS acronym can guide you before, during, and after eating. Practicing with these instructions can change the way you eat forever. It's the favorite takeaway of people who take my class.

> **B** stands for **Breathe and Belly Check Before You Eat.** Before you eat, take five deep breaths. Notice whether you have sensations of physical hunger, like mild gurgling or gnawing in the stomach. How hungry are you? What are you hungry for? Maybe you're hungry, or maybe you're bored, tired, or stressed. If you're physically hungry, take your time to choose food that you can enjoy and savor. If you're not, maybe there is something else your body is wanting, like movement or rest.

> **A** stands for **Assess your Food.** What does your food look like? Notice the colors. Does it look appealing? What

and taste, improves dental health, and spares your belly the discomfort of indigestion.

S stands for **Savor Your Food.** Food is a wonderful part of our lives. Savoring your food means a combination of the following: (1) taking time to choose food you really like and that would satisfy you right now, (2) picking food that honors your body *and* your taste buds, and (3) being fully present for the experience of eating and taking pleasure in that experience. Every time you sit down to eat can be an opportunity to savor.

Savoring Practice

Pick a time when you will be undisturbed, with no other distractions for about thirty minutes. Pick food that will be delicious and satisfying. It doesn't have to be a gourmet meal. For instance, I like nothing better than sitting down with a plate of fresh tomatoes (particularly in the summer), avocado, and goat cheese with some good balsamic vinegar and olive oil drizzled over the top, along with a few salty chips. Use the BASICS of Mindful Eating. Notice any time your mind wanders away from the experience of chewing, tasting, and savoring. It's okay that the mind wanders. Your job is just to notice and keep coming back to the experience of eating and savoring.

To support your practice, use the BASICS of Mindful Eating recorded meditation at http://www.LynnRossy.com/multimedia.

With practice, you can begin to hear the signs of belly hunger and distinguish it from the other times when you reach for food. This is an important step in understanding why, when, what, and how much to eat. Only by being in tune with your stomach and what it has to tell you can you establish balance between satisfying your body's need for food, your need for pleasure with food, and the other ways you can feed yourself without food.

Once you've determined that you are physically hungry and you begin to eat, how do you determine when to stop? Is it when the food is all gone? Or are there better ways of determining the amount of food to consume? If you've been in the clean-your-plate club for a long time, this will be a fun adventure. To honor your body, you will need to pay attention to stopping when your belly says "enough" as opposed to when the plate is empty.

Fullness is determined by the quantity of food you've eaten. If you have overeaten for a long time, this might be hard to determine, but it's not impossible to relearn. Tune in to differentiate between the sensations that your belly is no longer hungry but not yet full and the point of your belly feeling tight and uncomfortable. Between hunger and fullness there are many points when you can choose to stop eating. It's like putting gas into a car. You can be halfway full, three-quarters full, or completely full. Eating only until you are 80 percent full is practiced by certain cultures living in the "blue zones"—those places where people live the longest—so it's considered to contribute to better health and longevity.

One of the practices that will help you stop before you have eaten more than your body needs is to pick food that will satisfy

Savoring Practice

Whew! That's a lot to consider when you sit down to eat. Let's make it as simple as possible. Before you eat, ask yourself *Am I physically hungry?* If you're not, ask yourself why you're reaching for food. *Is there something else I need?* If you are hungry, ask *What would satisfy me at this meal? What food would help me feel energized and alive?* As you eat, check in with yourself throughout the meal to notice as you're getting full. Play around with stopping before you're all the way full—maybe 80 percent full. You will no longer feel hungry, but you won't yet feel full. While every meal doesn't need to be a scientific study, a little bit of attention to the changing bodily signals before and as you eat can lead to different choices as well as greater pleasure when you put fork to mouth.

food tastes? But it happens all the time. We are cut off from our sense of taste because we're lost in thought or engaged in some other activity. And many people rarely slow down enough to allow their attention to rest on the actual taste of the food they eat.

Take a moment to look, as if for the first time, at your food. Think about where it comes from. Reflect on the forces of nature that brought this food to life—the sunlight, the rain, the earth. As you eat, pay attention to the different tastes, textures, aromas, appearances of the food. Notice if the flavor stays with you after you chew and swallow or quickly disappears (usually a sign of more highly processed food). If you discover you don't like it, quit eating it. If you like it, take another bite, with full attention.

Paying attention in this way requires that you slow down. Reconnect with your senses and remember how this food is literally becoming you. Notice how the food transforms how you feel—for better or worse. All of these messages from your body can be your guide to how you eat in the future. Learning the wisdom of your body with each bite is how you connect your body, heart, mind, and belly in service of pleasure and health.

One bite, one taste, one smell can not only satisfy us in the present but create an explosion of memories of our past food experiences. The smell of bread baking always invites sweet memories of my mother baking bread. I always used to love to sneak under the damp kitchen towel covering the rising bread and sneak a pinch or two. I can still taste the stolen yeasty lump of dough melting in my mouth. Tasting pesto reminds me of picking basil in my garden and of all of the wonderful meals I've made with this savory sauce and

9.   A Breath Before You Tech

Slowing down in order to pay more careful attention to our lives can be accomplished in many ways, some quite creatively. For example, approximately 85 percent of you have a smartphone and use it regularly, so this next informal mindfulness practice will use this well-known technology to help us wake up and *really* connect instead of numbing out or distracting ourselves. What appears to be a wonderful tool to connect us with each other (the smartphone) has actually been shown to contribute to alienation from each other and from ourselves. As an act of freedom, we can choose to be aware of the endless interruptions that ring and vibrate through our days and turn them into moments of rest and true connection.

According to Deloitte's 2018 Global Mobile Consumer Survey it is estimated that the average consumer looks at their smartphone an average of fifty-two times every day! In a different survey, conducted by Asurion, even on vacation, four hours was the longest time that the average person studied could go before the need to check their phone became irresistible. In fact, this survey of two thousand people found that 31 percent feel regular anxiety at any point when separated from their phone, and 60 percent reported experiencing occasional stress when their phone is off or out of reach. Lastly (and this statistic might really surprise you), 62 percent would prefer to go *a week without chocolate* than lose their phone for just one day.

hand, take a deep breath and close your eyes. Continue to breathe deeply while you briefly scan your body for signs of tension or relaxation, coolness or warmth, energy or fatigue. Notice what you are feeling and thinking. Open your eyes and see what is in your surroundings. Are there sounds or smells available to you? Take a few more breaths to feel, hear, and experience all the senses available to you in this moment. After about fifteen seconds, decide what you'd like to do next. Maybe you want to check your phone, maybe you don't. Whatever you do, make it a conscious choice.

Make the practice even more profound by engaging in loving-kindness practice toward yourself during the pause. The instructions are pretty simple. While you're pausing, repeat to yourself *May I be safe. May I be happy. May I be healthy. May I live with joy and ease.* The practice of loving-kindness has been associated with higher vagal tone, representing an increase in the capacity for connection, friendship, and empathy as well as improved cardiovascular, glucose, and immune responses. Truly connect before you reach for the digital connect, then see how you feel.

More Savoring Practices: You can also decide to pause before you engage in other routine activities. Routine activities provide ample opportunities for us to use our mindfulness. You could pause and check in before you turn on the TV, while the computer is booting up, while you're waiting on hold for someone on the phone, while you're waiting at the red light, while you're waiting in line somewhere, or whenever you have a few seconds or minutes before an activity begins.

10. Do What's Important (Not Urgent)

Christophe Andre wrote in *Looking at Mindfulness: 25 Ways to Live in the Moment Through Art:* "Every day the things that are urgent in our lives come into conflict with those that are important." He goes on to add "If I don't do what's important, nothing will happen to me—at least not immediately. But gradually my life will become drab, sad, or strangely lacking in meaning." Since I read that, I have never looked at these two things—the urgent and the important—in the same way.

The very first time I noticed the tendency to take care of the urgent before the important, I was in my doctoral program studying psychology. I had a big test coming up, and I was pushing myself hard with the misguided belief that perfection was a possible and desirable goal. Feeling tired after studying for a few hours, I wanted to do some yoga. Then the thought, *You don't have time to do yoga! You need to keep studying!* hit me like a lightning bolt. I'm sure this type of thought had crossed my mind many times before, but this time I really heard it. It struck me how curious it was that I was learning to help other people take care of themselves better, yet I was using guilt to prevent myself from doing what I needed to do. Well, that was it. I have almost never again allowed the "urgent" to keep me from taking care of what's important—particularly when it comes to self-care!

wanting more (which is pretty unceasing!) even though you're not hungry, and you might decide it's more important to honor your belly. You can begin to experience the pleasure of listening to your body instead of the guilt and discomfort of eating more than it can handle easily.

If you don't do what's important, you might not notice for a while. But you will eventually begin to feel like the life you're living isn't your own. One meditation teacher called it "living an accidental life"—being pulled around by the constant flow of technology, activity, and demands of those around you as well as by the thoughts in your head. You might be either doing things to please someone else or meeting unreasonable expectations that you've set for yourself. However, when we take care of the important things in our life, we will be cultivating the relationships, self-care, and attention to purpose and meaning that truly feed our lives.

Right now, it is almost 3:15 p.m. and I am trying to decide whether to continue writing (I have given myself the goal of writing a thousand words a day) *or* go to yoga (something that I need in order to feel energized and calm). It's tricky, right? It could seem reasonable that I should tough it out and keep writing. How will I ever get a book written if I stop now? However, stepping back and taking the longer view, I realize if I don't take breaks to fill up my emotional, physical, and cognitive bank accounts, then I won't have anything to give. Having practiced meditation and yoga for many years, and knowing firsthand how essential they are for my well-being and my ability to get anything done that's worth doing, I will be going to yoga at 4:00 p.m.

Soothe (Instead of Eat) Your Emotions

Whatever the present moment contains, accept it as if you had chosen it. Always work with it, not against it.

—Eckhart Tolle

Reacting to emotions, from the difficult to the delightful, is one of the top reasons for overeating reported by people who come to my classes. Eating in reaction to difficult emotions—like sadness, anger, loneliness, boredom, stress, disappointment—reduces discomfort. Eating in reaction to delightful emotions—like happiness, joy, excitement—is a way to celebrate. Eating food in either instance is not inherently bad, but it's important to be compassionately conscious about when and how much you use eating as a strategy to manage emotions.

Particularly when difficult emotions arise, you have probably noticed that eating provides only *temporary* relief of the discomfort and *momentary* happiness. Eating as a solution becomes a set of new problems: feeling too full (sometimes when you weren't even physically hungry to begin with); experiencing shame (blaming yourself

11. Can You Name the Emotion?

When I teach meditation to beginners, I always start with a practice that guides people to notice their body's sensations, their feelings, and their thoughts. This investigation is not as easy as it
sounds. In fact, it is fairly common for people to say they find it
particularly difficult to identify the feeling that is present. This is
not surprising, for numerous reasons. Foremost, many of us were
taught as children to ignore or suppress our feelings. In my strict
upbringing, children were supposed to be seen but not heard.
Expressing your feelings was not encouraged and, to be fair, my
parents were also not educated in the world of emotions.

Before we go any further, let's first distinguish between emotions and feelings. While the two are quite related and used inter-
changeably all the time, they are technically different. Emotions
are responses occurring in the subcortical regions of the brain (spe-
cifically the amygdala, which is part of the limbic system). Emotions
are neurological reactions to a stimulus. For instance, when I'm
driving and a deer runs out in front of my car, I have the emotion
of fear. Fear, stemming from the fight-or-flight response, is like
other basic emotions; it is hard-wired in our bodies, is universal,
and is quite similar across humans.

Feelings, on the other hand, are the result of our awareness of
the emotions, coupled with our personal experiences, beliefs, memories, and thoughts—our individual conditioned perceptions. A
feeling is the result of your brain perceiving an emotion and your
assigning a certain meaning to it. While emotions are hard-wired,

sugar rush crashes, but I can also go out for a short walk, take a break to get a drink of water, or lie down for five minutes—all of which will energize me longer.

My friend Karen recently said, "When I start searching for sweets, I know something else is going on." This reaching for something to eat, even though you're not hungry, is a signal to pause and consider *What am I feeling?* Take time to name it. Notice what happens when you accurately label the feeling you're having. For me, it's kind of a relief. Like, *Oh, thanks for noticing.* If you choose to eat at this point, do so without guilt. But you might use this as an opportunity to understand yourself better and find that bringing compassion to yourself offers a kinder solution. Replacing emotional eating with the practice of naming your emotion can be an effective way of changing your patterns with food.

Sharon, a participant in my class, often experienced reaching for food when she felt overwhelmed and sad. After practicing for a few weeks, she shared that she was really benefiting from naming her emotion out loud to herself. "I'm noticing the feeling of being overwhelmed and I'm noticing the feeling of sadness." She allowed herself to feel them fully. Then, she profoundly stated, "I was so full of emotion, I had no room for food." So simple. So powerful.

Savoring Practice

Keep a journal to record your thoughts, feelings, and body sensations each day. It's particularly helpful to do this when you feel stressed, but you can also do it at less stressful times. For instance, you could

12. Feelings Are Natural, Mentionable, and Manageable

When we feel sad, lonely, afraid, ashamed, hopeless, anxious, and other difficult feelings, we can begin to feel like something has gone wrong. But feelings are not good or bad, right or wrong. Viewed through the lens of mindfulness, feelings are natural, mentionable, and manageable. Every feeling is a *naturally occurring* expression of our interaction with the world and the myriad inputs we receive moment by moment as well as the experiences and conditioning we have accumulated over a lifetime. When we experience a feeling, the first step is to *mention* it by name and to label it (as we discussed in the previous chapter). But often a deeper investigation is called for. When we experience difficult feelings, a mindfulness practice for *managing* them, called RAIN, can be useful for such an investigation.

RAIN is an acronym developed by Michele McDonald, a senior teacher of insight meditation, and widely used by mindfulness teachers around the world. RAIN stands for recognize, allow, investigate, and nonidentification or nurture. Tara Brach added "nurture" to the original practice to enhance your practice of self-compassion. This simple tool can help you work with discomfort and can be a substitute for reaching for food, alcohol, shopping, binge-watching TV, or other less-than-helpful activities that you might have used to soothe yourself when difficult feelings arise.

it's helpful to change the way you address the feeling. Instead of *I am angry*—which makes you the feeling—it is more helpful to say something like *anger is moving through me, anger is present, or I'm not anger; it is separate from me.* And then think of what you can do to *nurture* yourself in a healing way.

Let me give you an example. For a while after I got divorced, I would be home alone on the weekend, and I would notice feeling a little depressed. My reaction was to bake something, like cookies or brownies, because I love the smell of chocolate, and something hot out of the oven is so comforting. Knowing the acronym RAIN, instead of eating, I practiced with it as I felt the uncomfortable feelings.

R = Recognize. I recognized the feeling of loneliness.

A = Allow. *Loneliness is just what wants to be here right now.* I took a deep breath and allowed for the feeling to be present without judging it. Placing my hands over my heart helped me to do this.

I = Investigate. My body felt tired and sluggish. My feeling was loneliness. My story was *I'm lonely because I don't have any friends.* Then I would question, *Well, is that true?* Then I would count them on my fingers: *There is Althea, Sara, Nancy, Kim, Katherine, Laura, Martha, Jennifer, Peggy, Sarah...* When I had gotten up to ten, I stopped counting. It became obvious that the belief was incorrect. So I asked myself the obvious question: *If you're lonely, why don't you call one of your friends?* Answer: *I don't want to call one. Hmmm... then what is going on?* I kept looking and eventually I would

13. Feelings Times Three

One of the simplest ways to familiarize yourself with your feelings and understand them is to practice with the teaching from the second foundation of mindfulness. Through this lens, feelings are categorized three ways—they are either pleasant, unpleasant, or neither pleasant nor unpleasant (sometimes called *neutral*). As the teaching describes, every time we sense something through our eyes, ears, nose, mouth, body, or mind we experience (consciously or unconsciously) one of these three types of *feeling tones*.

Each feeling can result in a subsequent action or reaction, as follows:

1. If something is experienced as pleasant, you tend to want more of it (called *wanting*). Think about that first bite of chocolate cake or cold vanilla bean ice cream. It just calls out for *more*.

2. If something is experienced as unpleasant, you often want it to go away (called *aversion*). Think about the hurt of rejection or loneliness. You want it to go, so you try to push it away by fighting with it, distracting, or avoiding. Or you cover it up with the feeling of being fed and full.

3. If something is experienced as neutral, you tend to be confused about what is really going on (called *delu-sion*). Sometimes neutral is described by people as being *boring* because there isn't a strong feeling pulling

with cravings instead of compulsively acting on them. This strategy is fundamentally different from resisting, avoiding, or suppressing your feelings. Mindfulness teaches you to be aware of what is happening, create some space in which to evaluate the outcome of the different choices you could make, then choose your next step that aligns with compassionate care for yourself.

One of the most common statements I hear from people is "I can't stop eating, because it tastes so good!" However, when you know that pleasant sensations (and food) will always be available to you, then you don't need to act compulsively. You can discover, through experience, that it feels *more* pleasant to be fully present for your tasty food *and* stop eating before you get too full than it does to eat for pleasure until you're miserable.

You can also discover that you are resilient enough to feel an unpleasant sensation without needing to fix it, push it away, or eat it away. And you can discover that the many moments of neutral are actually preferable to the push and pull of pleasant and unpleasant.

Savoring Practice

But don't take my word for it. Discover for yourself whether this is true. When feelings arise, notice whether they are pleasant, unpleasant, or neutral. They can arise from something in the external environment (sounds, sights, and the like) or internally (emotions, thoughts, or body sensations). See if you can bring full awareness to the feelings without trying to change them. Where do you notice them in your body? What happens to the feelings over time? Watch as each feeling

14. Understanding the Five Hindrances

The five hindrances from the Buddhist teachings describe mental and emotional states that can overwhelm and confuse us. They can be examined during meditation or during the normal course of your day. These include desire (wanting), anger or aversion (not wanting), sleepiness, restlessness or worry, and doubt.

Desire

Desire shows up in the form of wanting what you don't have or more of what you do have. You might want more tasty food, more friends, more clothes, a better body, a different age, a newer car, or a bigger house. These desires are not bad. But many of them arise based on the messages that you get from ads, fads, and consumer culture about how you are supposed to be, how you are supposed to look, and how you are supposed to live. Using mindfulness, you can recognize when *wanting* is driving you (for example, to eat more just because it tastes so good) and watch your wanting instead of acting on it. On the other hand, skillful (or helpful) desire can arise in the form of wanting to be your best self.

Anger and Aversion

Aversion is wanting things to be different from how they are, and anger can arise toward anyone or anything that is in the way of

Restlessness and Worry

When I ask people what they notice after meditation practice, the most common responses I hear are "I was thinking about my to-do list" or "I was thinking about all of the things I need to get done." Obviously, they are pointing at the same thing—concern about the future. Worry and anxiety arise from the fear of not getting it all done, having it turn out bad, or having things go wrong.

Restlessness can also be the result of not getting enough movement into your day, particularly if you have a sedentary job. Or if you fuel yourself regularly with coffee and other caffeinated drinks and food, this can bring on restlessness. And sometimes restlessness arises in response to a difficult feeling you'd rather avoid.

Doubt

Doubt can be present when you are caught in confusion, indecision, uncertainty, and lack of confidence. Doubt often makes it hard for you to act on a decision; it can lead you to question your ability. Doubt is a trickier hindrance to recognize because you get so caught up in the indecision that you don't realize it is happening.

For instance, doubt can lead to questioning how mindful eating can ever help you. You can convince yourself that it isn't working. Doubt then becomes a self-fulfilling prophecy. The more doubt stops you from practicing, the less effective it will become. Then you convince yourself it is the practice that isn't working, not the fact that you are not engaging it in. Oh, yes; doubt is very tricky.

When restlessness or worry arise, make deep breathing your first responder. This will reverse the fight-or-flight response. Plus, by focusing on breathing, you have much less attention available for the thoughts and beliefs that are fueling your worries.

When doubt arises, question it. What are your beliefs, thoughts, stories, feelings, fears, and anxieties about the situation? What would happen if you decided to try something new or decided on a path? Some people are more prone to doubt than others. Work on making small decisions and taking small steps when you can. Celebrate the small victories over doubt.

The next time you feel upset and a subsequent snacking urge arises, start by tapping into the power of healing, compassionate self-touch.

A common compassion practice is placing your hands over your heart. This gesture is especially comforting when you are experiencing challenging emotions or you are in the presence of someone else who is having difficulty. It's pretty simple. When you notice strong emotions, place your hands over your heart. Feel the touch and warmth of your hands on your chest, and let your hands rest with the gentle expansion and deflation of the chest as you breathe. Deepen the breath slightly to counteract some of the stress you are feeling.

While your hands are resting on your chest, it can be helpful to imagine breathing in the qualities that would benefit you right now—safety, acceptance, love, kindness, contentment. Breathe in a sense of ease and peace. Breathe out anything you want to let go of. Breathe in a caring feeling of self-love and compassion. Breathe out any self-loathing or limiting thoughts that might be present. Spend a few moments here and feel the touch of your hands on your heart. Spend as much time here as you would like until you notice a softening of your body and release of tension.

The experience of being touched is vital to life, just like eating. If you eat three meals a day, try giving yourself three hugs or kind touches a day. Hug other people (after getting permission, of course!) whenever you can. You increase your touch quotient, and you help the people around you feel the love.

3. Rub your hands together vigorously for fifteen seconds and then close your eyes. Cup your warm hands over both eyes for a few more seconds and sense your face beginning to relax and soften.

4. Place your hands over a part of your body that you commonly judge harshly. Send love and acceptance through your hands to this part of your body as best you can. If thoughts of judgment arise, notice them and let them go. Say to your body *I love and accept you just as you are, I am your friend and I want to take care of you,* or other statements that bring kindness and compassion to your body.

To support your practice, use the *Healing with Self-Touch* recorded meditation at http://www.LynnRossy.com/multimedia.

feel an emotional connection, but you don't hang on to them. You watch with some distance. In general, once the movie is over, so are the feelings.

You can do the same with yourself. Notice and experience everything like you're watching a movie—without having to change it, chase it, push it away, or avoid it. Allow feelings to come and go. Enjoy the pleasant while it's here, don't worry so much about the unpleasant when it arises, and when things are neutral, enjoy the experience of calm.

Another practice, called *urge surfing,* was developed by Dr. Alan Marlatt to help prevent relapse from addiction treatment. View your urges to drink, overeat, or binge snack as if they are waves in the ocean that arise, peak, and eventually break on the shore and retreat. This way of viewing urges uses the understanding of impermanence as an aid to be with the passing body sensations, thoughts, and emotions without acting on them.

Breathing with the wave cycle of emotions can be used as an alternative to comfort eating and other behaviors that are only temporarily satisfying. You can pay attention to urges or cravings to eat in the absence of hunger (whether for emotional or environmental reasons), then breathe with the wave of the urge without eating. See how long the urge lasts if you don't give in to it. Often people in my mindful eating classes tell me that if they stop to notice the urge, it passes quite quickly or they forget about it altogether.

However, not all urges will be equal in size, strength, or frequency. I have read that urges last anywhere from two to thirty minutes, but rarely longer than thirty minutes if you are actively working to ride them out instead of fighting with them. Urges will

17. Healing with Movement

Many people tend to be like walking heads—disconnected from their bodies from the neck down. Living too much in the top floor (the head) is often associated with dwelling on obsessive, negative, and ruminative thoughts. This kind of time spent in your head rarely solves your problems or soothes your emotions. However, by dropping down into the rest of your body and placing your attention on the sensations below your neck, you take the attention away from the thoughts that are creating despair.

When you are stressed, angry, sad, afraid, lonely, or confused, how often do you find yourself sitting around listening to the thoughts spinning out in your head—maybe even while you head to the kitchen for something to eat? While there is a time and place for sitting mindfully with your thoughts and feelings, you can also employ the enormously helpful strategy of moving your body. Physical movement can provide tremendous emotional relief as well as important physical benefits.

Think of physical movement as both a preventative strategy and a prescription for whenever you are feeling down. If you can start making physical activity a part of your daily life, then, when you really need a boost, you are more likely to remember how good you feel when you move. Whether you like to put down the yoga mat, put on the running shoes, jump on a bike, jump in the pool, or take a brisk walk, physical activity has been shown to reduce symptoms of anxiety, depression, and stress as well as increase your motivation and energy. In fact, physical activity has been shown to be as

Savoring Practice

Start by scanning your body and notice any aches or pains as well as places of comfort and peace. Begin to breathe a little more deeply. See if you can intuit what your body would most like to do right now. When you are ready, begin to stretch in a way that would feel supportive. Take your time and take it slow. You might move your head from side to side to stretch your neck, you might roll your shoulders, you might bring your arms up overhead and stretch toward the clouds. Move and notice what happens. Breathe deeply through every movement. And let your body guide you.

If you're a little unsure of what to do, that's okay. The more you pay attention, the more you will be able to respond lovingly to your body and determine what it needs. The most important thing to remember is to be present with kindness. Let it be a time when you are communing with yourself without judgment and living beyond the stories in your head.

More Savoring Practices: I believe that yoga practice is one of the most healing activities that you can do. If you're a little hesitant to go to a class, try the yoga videos on my website at http://www.lynnrossy. com/multimedia. There are floor, standing, and chair versions. These have been used by people around the world to reduce pain and increase a sense of well-being. Yoga is one of the best ways to create a positive, loving relationship to your body. Remember, it's the only body you have. Treat it well.

of living—one that doesn't need the extra layer of drama or the extra donut in order to feel okay. Training yourself to look more closely at the present moment, you can begin to soften and relax into an examination of your senses, which are constantly in flux. Every nanosecond, experience changes. (A nanosecond is one-billionth of a second. That's a lot of stuff happening all of the time!)

I have spent a lot of time paying mindful attention to what is happening in the present moment. There are immeasurable sounds, sights, smells, touches, and tastes to experience that can keep you from being bored. Equally important is that each moment we are alive can be viewed as an incredible miracle. When we see the present moment clearly, we get in touch with the amazing wonder of living in a body and even the blessing of each breath. Mindful eating, in particular, is an experience filled with delicious morsels that could keep you from being bored, even when you are eating alone.

This doesn't mean that you just sit around all day. But I am suggesting that you spend some time each day *just being*, without distractions, and with a degree of curiosity that changes the boring to the fascinating. Look carefully at the thing you call boring to see what is really going on. Boredom is simply a lack of attention. Is there tension in your body? Is there an uneasiness about what to do? Is there a story that says you should be working all of the time? Is there a belief that more is always better? Is there something driving you? And if so, what is it?

Instead of assuming that you have to constantly strive or be entertained, be willing to examine carefully whether this is absolutely true. Reflect on whether striving is creating positive

and come back to sitting, breathing, seeing, hearing. Repeatedly reminding yourself to relax helps to facilitate a letting go. After a couple of minutes, notice what happens to the striving. Does it increase or decrease? Is there a greater or lesser sense of calm? While it might not happen in the first or even second sitting, most people begin to experience the shift from feeling bored to an increased ability to find the wonder in the present moment that needs no extra excitement or stimulation...or second helpings.

or some type of uneasiness, this is the time to listen and determine what choices to make. On the other hand, when your body is at ease and your heart feels open, you are receiving the message that you are operating in sync with your body's needs.

Unfortunately, when we have an ache or pain (physical or emotional) we tend to respond in ways that create more dis-ease. This happens when you resort to drinking too much caffeine when you're tired, eating too much food when you're feeling stressed or sad, taking too much medication or drinking too much alcohol when you're upset, and overworking and getting busier in order to run away from something you don't want to feel. These actions tell your body that you're not listening and that you don't care. You numb yourself, distract yourself, and self-medicate under the false belief that this will help. But your attempts will only lead to more pain, rather than less. What all of these strategies have in common is a lack of kind presence and care.

Alternatively, when you feel discomfort in your body, an increase in your curious awareness of what is happening might require you to feel the pain, but ultimately it gives you a roadmap to feeling better. All you have to do is pause and take a breath. Ask yourself, *What is my body trying to tell me? What do I need to learn?* Listen for a minute and hear the messages that arise. You might hear something as simple as *get some rest* or *get moving*. It might be something more involved, having to do with a relationship or a work situation that you haven't been addressing.

Let's take this conversation to the area of eating. What does your body tell you about how you feed it? Your body naturally would like to feel energized, alert, and strong. So it asks for foods

perceptions in your mind. There is a direct feedback loop from what it is experiencing to the messages it sends.

Experience the joy of giving your body what it wants. Instead of working against your body, with practice you can discover that there is nothing more pleasurable than being a compassionate partner with your entire being—body, heart, and mind. Feed, move, and live in ways that show your body you love it, and it will respond with energy, joy, and ease.

need some couples counseling with yourself. Or, at the very least, a big modification in your relationship is in order.

One day I was beating myself up about not doing something perfectly enough, and my husband, overhearing me, said "Don't talk to my best friend like that." This statement stopped me in my tracks. First of all, it was very sweet. And second, it really made me stop and consider what I was doing. Why wasn't I being my own best friend? Although I had already spent years examining my negative beliefs about myself, there was obviously still work to be done.

In a wonderful poem by the fourteenth century poet Hafiz, he says "Now is the time to know that your every thought is holy." This means that every thought you encourage and feed has an effect on your body, heart, and mind. And because of that, it is of great importance. When you pause to consider the significance of this truth, I hope you realize that it's time to make a lasting truce with yourself and try expressing love as the only reasonable option.

In the same vein, Louise Hay wrote, "Remember, you have been criticizing yourself for years and it hasn't worked. Try approving of yourself and see what happens." If that's still a new concept for you, it might help to consider the reasons for treating yourself with anything but respect. Much of the tyranny comes from past conditioning by others (such as family, friends, peers) and a culture that thrives on having us think less of ourselves. Consider the effect that negativity has had on your life. For me, the effect was to suck all of the joy out of it, and at some point I just said "Enough!" How about you? Are you ready to make a truce with yourself? Are you ready to make peace with food and your body? Have you had "enough" of your own negativity? I hope so.

sluggish, unwell, and overfull. I probably won't be perfect at it, but please be patient with me as I vow to create new patterns of kindness and compassion toward you. I will do my best to give you the right food, sleep, movement, play, and anything else you need to operate at your best and to know that you are loved.

With deepest sincerity and love,

Lynn

Note: Because habits are hard to break, you will continue to hear the negative voices in your head. Instead of reacting to their presence, work on changing the storyline. If you need more help with this, read on. The next section is all about surrendering limiting beliefs.

Surrender Limiting Thoughts

Nothing can harm you as much as your own thoughts unguarded.

—Buddha

It's been estimated that we have between thirty-five and forty-eight thoughts per minute (or fifty thousand to seventy thousand thoughts per day), and most of them are negative, repetitive, and false. These "automatic thoughts" arise out of nowhere, exist, and pass away, over and over again throughout the course of the day, and they often wreak emotional havoc on the uninitiated. The uninitiated to mindfulness, that is. Without an understanding of how to listen and respond to the thoughts in your head, you can often feel at their mercy. Mindfulness teaches you how to be with thoughts without becoming them. You can see their patterns and behaviors and transform them through your loving awareness.

Unfortunately, most of us were never taught how to be aware of our thought patterns—or that there was anything we could do about them. Well, don't worry. In this step, I list the common thoughts that I hear from participants in my classes about their

21. The Paradox of Acceptance and Change

I can't love myself until I change _____ (fill in the blank: weigh less, fit into a smaller size, be less wrinkled, look the way I did twenty years ago). Sound like a familiar limiting thought? You are bombarded with both subliminal and overt messages from social media, advertising, movies, television, the diet industry, and sometimes even friends and family that you need to change in order to be lovable.

The corporate world makes money only if you think you need to change. Making you feel less than worthy is what they count on to get you to buy their products. The strategy of Hollywood is to make unachievable and unnatural (airbrushed and surgically altered) images seem attractive so that you will idolize their heroes and heroines and want to become like them. Friends and family might be more well-intentioned, but their messages often come from their own discomfort about themselves and their lack of understanding of how love is truly expressed and help is offered. For instance, Emily told me that she remembers her father telling her at age five, when she was in the kitchen for bread and butter (her favorite snack), "You better stop eating or no man will ever marry you!"

Any message saying you need to be different in order to feel good about yourself does nothing to help you and a lot to hurt you. In fact, there is substantial evidence of a worldwide prevalence of body image dissatisfaction and its negative impact on psychological you treat yourself as an adversary, you are likely to fail. But when you become your own best friend, you want to treat yourself well. Developing a friendly and caring relationship with yourself is a loving journey that is much more likely to help you achieve any goals that you might have.

Consider that the foundation for everything else in your life flows from the quality of the relationship you have with yourself. If you treat yourself with love, respect, and compassion, you will partner with yourself to achieve the things that have meaning to you. If you treat yourself with criticism, disapproval, disdain, or indifference, you'll tend to shut down and engage in self-defeating behaviors.

The paradox of acceptance and change is that you love yourself first, flaws and all—even your tendency to overeat or emotionally soothe with food. In this way, you have already won. While you don't *need* to change, if changes to the way you eat could make you happier, healthier, or more fulfilled, then you can change while you're loving yourself. In fact, through loving yourself you will be spending less energy on negativity and more energy on the things that make a positive difference, like trying out some new recipes, taking a cooking class, learning how to dance, or engaging in a new pastime. The list is endless.

Savoring Practice

If the mantra you have had up until now has been anything like "I'm not okay the way I am," then it's time to try a new one. In the yoga tradition, mantras (words or statements repeated over and over) are used to

22. Understanding the Wanting Mind

Hands down, the most frequent response I get from people about why they overeat is "It tastes so good; I can't stop." And, who can blame them, right? If you are eating a wonderful dish of peach cobbler à la mode and it tastes delicious, you want to keep eating. You don't want to leave a morsel of peach (or the ice cream that's on top of it!) on the plate. The taste buds are singing—"Yummmmm!" Then the taste buds partner with the mind, and this is when the trouble ensues. The mind doesn't seem to know when to stop.

We tend to live at the mercy of what I call the *wanting mind*. The wanting mind seeks pleasure as its main occupation—its secondary occupation being to avoid pain. Of course, it makes sense psychologically that we want more of the things that are pleasant and less of the things that are unpleasant in our lives. Every day, often quite unknowingly, you make an inordinate number of decisions based on this principle. This principle can influence how much you eat, how you dress, where you live, who you spend time with, how you spend your time, how you spend your money, and so much more. However, this constant activity of seeking pleasure and avoiding pain can have a definite downside. In the case of the peach cobbler, for instance, you might end up being completely stuffed.

So let's break this down a bit. When you are eating, it is important to consider both your taste buds and your belly. Paying attention to the sensations of taste by mindfully attending to what you understand the idea of stopping while there is still food, so we have to remember that there is more to consider than the immediate gratification of how something tastes in the moment. There is the longer-term gratification of having less indigestion and fatigue as a result of not overeating.

Knowing and respecting your patterns and triggers with food will help you better understand the times, places, and situations that might get in the way of your succeeding at stopping before you're stuffed when something tastes good. For example, if you know that bringing home a gallon of ice cream is a disaster waiting to happen, don't do that. Instead, go to the ice cream parlor and get a cup or cone. Sit down and really savor it. Know that you can always come back and get ice cream again when you want it.

Savoring Practice

What is one food that you overeat because "it tastes so good"? Set aside a time to eat it as an experiment. Before you eat, ask your *body* how much would be "enough." Portion out the amount that your belly (not your mind) wants, and put it on a plate or in a dish. Of course, be aware that your mind might have its own opinion (hint: it will probably want more). Be sure to have no other distractions: just eat, and savor your pleasurable food. Take your time. Chew each bite thoroughly. Breathe between mouthfuls. After each mouthful, notice how you feel. Try stopping when your belly (not your mind) has had enough.

23. Food Is Just Food

The limiting thought *There's good food and bad food* is a type of all-or-nothing thinking common to people in my mindful eating classes. The idea of putting food into categories of "good" and "bad" has been programmed into our brains by the diet culture and the food industry whose products promote the latest food fads. For instance, low-fat products have been promoted for years because fat was considered "bad." Now the keto diet tells you fat is "good," and keto food products have become mainstream. You can see and hear the ever-changing diet declarations promoted in the grocery aisles, the book club, the gym, the moms' group, during cocktail hour, and anywhere else where people are gathered. The next step? You put *yourself* into the category of being "good" or "bad" based on which foods you did or didn't eat.

How does this show up in the life of an eater? Joan said that she was working hard one day, with back-to-back meetings, and she found herself in the middle of the afternoon feeling like she wanted a break. Joan had been taking my Eat for Life class, so she had learned to check in with herself to see what she really needed in these moments. *What am I really hungry for?* she asked herself. She might have discovered that she needed to take a walk around the block, get a glass of water, or do a few yoga moves. However, after pausing and giving herself time to reflect, the answer she received was *a chocolate chip cookie.* From experience she had learned to question food as the ultimate answer at such times, so she checked in again. *What are you really hungry for, dear?* Again, the specific answer

There could be a number of outcomes to this story. Joan could have felt so bad that she didn't have the cookie at all. She could have reacted to the harshness of the restrictive voice, said, *Screw it,* and bought a dozen cookies and begun to plow through them (see more on this pattern in the next chapter). She might have bought one but known she was being watched by the "food police" so she ate it so fast that she didn't really enjoy it. Or Joan could have recognized the "cookies are bad" thoughts for what they are—just thoughts. In this last scenario, Joan could have had her cookie and enjoyed it too.

And what did Joan do? I'm happy to say that Joan was able to catch herself in the tennis match of thoughts and knew that it is okay to have a cookie. She bought her cookie and savored it with great delight. It was what she wanted, and she was happy that she had learned to listen to herself.

This does not mean that every afternoon Joan needs a chocolate chip cookie. Other days she finds that she wants to do something else to refresh her body and mind. Life without the answers already pinned down gives you the freedom to discover your own knowing about what is the most skillful action to take. Living life in the middle, without the extremes, takes a little more attention, kindness, curiosity, and time, but it allows for the sweetness of life to be embraced in each moment, even if it shows up in the form of a chocolate chip cookie.

Breaking out of the prison of good and bad requires a mind-set change. First of all, it's important that you know you can have anything that you want. There is no good or bad food, and you are not good or bad based on what you eat. Second, you can decide that

24. Taking Care of Your Two-Year-Old Self

From inside, do you ever scream, *I'll eat as much as I want to! Watch me!*? Living under the scrutiny of *good* and *bad, should* and *shouldn't, ought to* and *ought not, must* and *must not* will eventually result in a pattern of thinking and behavior that is hurtful and self-sabotaging. I call it *the revenge of the two-year-old.*

Think about how a two-year-old acts and behaves. They call it the "terrible twos" because this age group wants a say in what they eat and do instead of following the expectations and rules they hear from their parents. "No! You can't tell me what to do" is a common declaration you will hear from the mouths of these adorable little babes.

The same thing happens to you when you have heard quite enough of the reprimands and rules about how to eat perfectly in every moment. When the rules or scolding become too onerous, the common and understandable reaction is to throw a little fit and go out of control in defiance. The inner toddler ends up crying, and you end up eating more than you really want. And you seldom end up feeling better as a result. A toddler, at least, is moving through an important developmental stage, but you, as an adult, are just left with the feeling of desperation, shame, guilt, and being overly full!

Because the rule maker is so common in us, due to the influence of the diet culture, I am pretty confident that you have had the experience of both setting up food rules and then acting rebellious peace with food. She was stuck in the "I'm going to eat whatever I want!" stage that was tinged with agitation, instead of a calmer acknowledgment that "I *can* have whatever I want and mindfully choose what and how much that is." Can you sense the difference in the two similar but very different statements?

Over the course of ten weeks, Jenny began to use mindfulness to taste her food with greater awareness and feel her fullness signals with more kindness and compassion. Instead of simply reacting based on past conditioning, she was learning to access the information available to her in the present moment to determine the choices she would make. Even though at the beginning of class her resignation was palpable, her budding ability to be present with each eating experience, using a beginner's mind, helped her to move out of resistance and into a softer attitude toward food.

In week ten, Jenny shared that her journey with food had been mainly about leaving behind both the rules and the reaction to the rules so that she could have an authentic, loving relationship with herself, her body, and the food that she eats.

I know that if I take a couple of deep breaths before I eat and let the competing voices in my head arise and pass away, I am able to feel deeply into what I need most in the moment. Sometimes I want the food that I see in front of me, and sometimes I actually decide I need something different. It feels nice to sense what my adult decision would be and act on it accordingly. I let the two-year-old me know that she can always have tasty goodies, but there are other activities we can enjoy together as well.

25. Moving Past the Scarcity Mentality

"How do you know when it's time to stop eating?" I ask.

"I can't quit eating until my plate is empty" is the common response.

It shouldn't be too hard to grasp how this "clean your plate" strategy might be problematic. Most fundamentally, this approach completely ignores your belly and the signs of fullness—the most natural and beneficial indicator of when to stop eating. How did we go so astray?

To start, as a child you probably heard your mother tell you to clean your plate because there are starving children somewhere in the world. Not that any of those children will receive the food you don't eat, by the way. Although not being wasteful is an important lesson to learn, when it entails forcing children to eat beyond their fullness signals it is misguided. This teaches children that their own natural signals to stop eating are to be ignored. And this can be pinpointed as a time when many children stop listening to their bodies for guidance.

At a wellness conference a few years back, I spoke about the strategy of stopping when you're full—not when there is no more food on the plate—and the practice of saving the leftover food for later *or* throwing away a few bites as you learn how much your body needs. Surprisingly, there were dietitians who were just as

I also want to acknowledge that wasting food is tragic, considering that one in six American children lives in a state of food insecurity—not knowing where their next meal will come from—and 821 million people suffer from hunger worldwide. And waste we do. Somewhere between 30 and 40 percent of the United States' food supply is wasted. But when you spend a little time discovering how much your body really needs through mindful investigation, you will actually waste less by serving yourself less, not needing to throw saved food away because it has spoiled, and not treating your body like a waste can.

A poster from the World War II era tells the story of "Waste No Food." In a lengthy exposé, the poster says food is wasted "when too much is served at a meal, when too much is prepared for a meal, when burned or spoiled in cooking, and when handled carelessly." Notably, at the bottom of the poster in bold letters it says "Food is wasted when we eat more than our bodies need for growth and repair and to supply energy for our work."

Nowhere does it say to clean your plate or eat more than your body needs. But these informative posters do give a lot of other alternatives to wasting food (see below). While it might take a little more time and effort, teaching *these* ethics and practices to your children (and practicing them yourself) will truly benefit the world.

In deciding when it's time to push the plate away, the French (famous for not overeating) have been shown to respond to different eating signals from the ones Americans heed. In one study, 133 participants from Paris and 145 from Chicago were asked to complete a brief survey on their food habits, including questions on how

More Savoring Practices: If I've inspired you, and you want to explore more waste-avoiding strategies that are much more beneficial than eating what your body doesn't need, here are some ideas.

- Store food so that it doesn't spoil.

- Actually use leftovers.

- Buy local.

- Grow your own food.

- Create a compost pile or worm bin.

- Enjoy vegetarian or vegan meals at least one day a week.

- Donate to food banks.

- Freeze fruits and vegetables.

- Learn to can and preserve.

- Blend your leftover vegetables and ripening fruit.

- Use your coffee grounds as a fertilizer.

- Plan your meals.

- Take your lunch.

- Cook at home.

- Buy whole foods.

being aware of reaching for food and putting it into their mouths. Eating is a routine activity, and food is abundantly available. When we travel on airplanes, my husband asks me to take the cookies and pretzels away from him before he finds his hand throwing the food into his mouth. We are a little like robots: *See food. Eat food.*

My husband listens to me talk about mindful eating all of the time, so he is aware of the temptation of food sitting on his tray table. However, we are generally unaware of all of the food-related decisions we make on a daily basis—many due to external factors in the environment (like stewardesses handing us snacks!). For instance, if you are given a larger serving, you will tend to eat more. If the food is convenient and visible, you are more likely to reach for it. Dim, softer lighting in a room promotes eating for longer periods of time. The type of label on a packaged food influences whether you want it. And the list goes on. In fact, it is estimated that we make more than two hundred food-related decisions a day, which often lead to unconsciously eating without considering what or how much we select and consume.

Savoring Practice

Five different types of food-related decisions have been proposed, based on *when, what, how much, where,* and *who.* Let's use those to create some mindfulness practices that might break you out of a robotic way of eating and into the world of conscious eating.

When: How do you decide *when* to eat? Do you eat when you're hungry or just when food is available or you're feeling

- When waking up to the next bite, part of your consideration might be *where* and how the food was produced. Notice the difference in how nourished and satisfied you feel, between eating food from a local farmer and food shipped from far away.

Who: Consider the influence of the people around you in how you eat. At home and work, who is influencing you for the better or worse? Who encourages you to eat in a way that you like to eat? Who encourages you to eat in a way that you *don't* like to eat? How can you spend more time with those who have your best self in mind rather than those that don't? Who you keep company with can make a big difference in how you eat.

Attention: To give yourself loving attention, pay attention to the *triangle of awareness*—feelings, thoughts, and body sensations. These messages can help you learn to respond to your needs more directly and effectively.

Acceptance: It can be hard to give yourself attention if you lack self-acceptance. In fact, the spotlight on yourself can often reveal negative self-talk and behaviors. Working on the steps toward self-acceptance can boost your self-confidence and self-worth. And until you give it to yourself, it is difficult to receive it from others.

Appreciation: Appreciation is really at the heart of using food as reward. One of our deepest needs is to be seen and appreciated. When you don't feel acknowledged and appreciated for the things that you accomplish or just for who you are, you can look to other methods for your hit of endorphins. Don't wait for something or someone else to give you appreciation. In one of the movement practices that I teach, I end with having people pat themselves on the shoulders as they say "Good job!" It always brings a smile and a softening of tension.

Affection: Affection requires the preceding three keys, but it also involves some behavior that demonstrates it—in other words, affection is conveyed, is manifested by actions. A display of affection grows out of loving attention, self-acceptance, and appreciation. Affection fosters a sense of safety and inspires caring actions.

Acceptance: Remind yourself of the perfection of your imperfection every day. At least once a day, when you look in the mirror, say "I love you" and smile. It's like taking your daily love potion.

Appreciation: As you go through your day, pay attention to the accomplishments you feel good about. Don't ignore the little moments of feeling satisfied—making your bed in the morning, getting the dishes done, getting the kids off to school, getting to work on time, writing an email that accomplished a goal, getting dinner on the table, making it to the post office in time to get a package into the mail, and so on. These small moments make up your life.

Affection: Show yourself affection every day by engaging in small random acts of kindness toward yourself. These acts can include fixing yourself a cup of tea and relaxing for a couple of minutes in the middle of a busy day, feeding yourself nourishing food when you're hungry, taking a short walk, pausing and taking five long deep breaths, placing your hands over your heart and connecting with your feelings, getting a massage, taking a hot bath with candles, taking a restorative yoga class, taking a mini-nap, and many more.

Allowing: Perhaps the biggest reward is this: "I completely and fully love and appreciate myself for every aspect of my being." This statement or one like it can be the touchstone to bring you into skillful relationship with yourself. Develop your own declaration of worth and write it down so that you can read it and reflect on it regularly.

hands over her heart and breathe in the memory of her connection with her mother and sister. Although she had lost them from the physical world, her memory of them could support and comfort her when she took the time to stop and feel into the truth of their love, untarnished and unbroken by death.

Mark used the belief that he was "bored" as a way of using food and media to entertain him and distract him from the underlying issue of loneliness. In the last class, Mark reported that he had connected with a meetup group of like-minded individuals and reported he was going out on a date. He said, "I thought I needed to lose weight before I could date. But now I know that was just an excuse because I was scared to put myself out there. Now I'm ready to face my fears with the knowledge that I'm good enough to be someone's friend."

There is practically no effort required in finding and eating food—it's ubiquitous, fast, and easy. But looking to food for comfort is like settling for a bad boy- or girlfriend. They both promise more than they can give and leave you feeling worse than when you started out. The courage to face your fears and desires will challenge you and demand that you dig a little deeper and feel a little more. When you don't settle for quick fixes (or bad dating choices), you have the chance to change the narrative, connect with your own resilience, and meet your real needs. Understanding what lies underneath your habit of reaching for food for comfort or entertainment takes a little extra effort—and you're worth it!

29. There Is No Success or Failure

"I've already blown it, so I might as well keep on eating and start fresh tomorrow." Karen is describing how she sabotages herself. "Then tomorrow comes and I do the same thing over again. I set myself up to fail by setting unrealistic goals, and then I eat more than I really want because I say I'm never going to do it again."

Perfectionism, and related defeatism, are at the heart of this faulty thinking. When eating is measured by elusive, confusing, impossible-to-live-by rules, you are destined to fail on a regular basis. Feeling defeated is an understandable consequence.

In the back of her mind, Karen had many of the common ideas about the "right" and the "wrong" ways to eat, based on what she'd read and heard from others. The rules were sometimes vague and often ephemeral, due to how frequently dieting advice changes. "But somehow," Karen reflected, "I just know I'm not doing it right." If you're like Karen, all it takes is eating one blameless piece of cake or innocent piece of chocolate, and you've failed—even more, you're a failure.

The good news is there is no "good" or "bad," "right" or "wrong," "success" or "failure" on the journey of mindful eating. And thank goodness! What a dreary world it would be if success lay in never eating chocolate (or other maligned goodies) again! The "rules" of mindful eating entail paying attention, with kindness and curiosity, to all of the flavors, sights, smells, and other senses available to you *without judgment*. Yes, you do cultivate clarity about the failed. Have your donut, or whatever else it is you want, with full attention to the taste and without the extra icing of guilt. It tastes so much better that way! And if your "Betty" shows up to shame you, thank her for sharing and ask her to sit down and have a cup of tea while you're enjoying yourself. Who knows? She might even join you for a donut!

In truth, that perfectionist part of you developed when you were a child in order to protect you in some way. For me, I believe it was formed, in part, as a way of helping myself "be perfect" so that my dad would be happy. When we're children, we think the world revolves around us and whatever is going on must be our fault. *Dad's dark mood must have been my fault,* I thought. If I was just good enough, Dad would feel better. While it didn't work, the part was formed and followed me into adulthood.

The work as an adult is to befriend the critical, perfectionist thoughts in your head. It's the reaction to the thoughts in your head that keep them active and perpetual. But when you learn not to react to the snarky voice in your head criticizing you, then it becomes a little confused. *What, no reaction?* said my Betty. *What's the fun of that?* Over time, the voice becomes much more manageable and much less frequent.

Savoring Practice

If perfection has been your goal, then my guess is you have rarely, if ever, succeeded. To err is human. So relax and join the human race with the rest of us. It's okay. In fact, it is more than okay. It is preferable and

30. Well-Being Has No Size

Lynda seemed pretty agitated when I picked her up to go to the gym one morning. When asked what was going on, she explained that she desperately wanted to lose weight before a reunion of college girlfriends she hadn't seen in a long time. She had been trying to work out more and eat better, but her weight wasn't changing.

"I'm so frustrated. I'm never going to lose weight" is a limiting observation I hear over and over again. Sound familiar?

People often use special events like reunions and weddings as a reason to try to lose weight and "look good." This strategy doesn't work very often, and even if it does, the weight comes back and often even more after the event—an unfortunate reality of quick-weight-loss schemes.

The mind-set is *I need to be different in order to be okay* and *I'm not enough the way I am.* This mind-set that can keep you from exploring well-being and how it's uniquely achieved in your life. It's a mind-set that will create suffering for you, regardless of whether you lose weight or not. Even if you get to a "magic number" that you think will make you happy, you will quickly find some other way you need to change in order to be okay.

I discovered this many years ago during my recovery from drugs, alcohol, and cigarettes. Cigarettes were my last big addiction, and when I finally quit, I became quite depressed, ate a lot of ice cream and brownies, and gained quite a bit of weight. During the years of diet attempts that followed, I decided that I needed to

Savoring Practice

Using those four categories, take a few minutes to reflect and write down the types of activities that produce a sense of well-being in your life.

Under *physical movement,* write down the types of activities that you enjoy, who you like to enjoy them with, when you can make time for them, and where you like to do them.

Under *emotional connection,* write down the people whom you'd like to spend more time with—those who are like-minded, supportive, loyal, interesting, trustworthy, dependable, and positive. (Of course, you can't expect all your needs to be met with one person—that's totally impossible!—and not every person will have every quality.) Plan for time in the next week with someone on your list.

Under *mental stimulation and creativity,* write down as many activities and pursuits as you can think of that would interest you in the areas of education, occupation, social engagement, and leisure (think classes, workshops, reading, arts like painting and music, podcasts, cooking, traveling, puzzles).

Under *spiritual expression,* write down the ways that you feel a greater sense of connection and peace (spending time in nature, engaging with a particular religious or spiritual community, readings on relevant topics, meditating, doing yoga).

Be as specific as possible in each of the categories and visualize yourself being the person who meets these needs. In fact, start to schedule in time for the activities and people that most resonate with your heart.

Smile and Create Your Own Happiness

Be happy in the moment, that's enough. Each moment is all we need, not more.

—Mother Teresa

Now that you are learning to slow down, soothe your emotions, and surrender limiting beliefs, you are perfectly prepared to add the next step—smile and create your own happiness. People are often surprised when I tell them that mindfulness is not just about being present; it also includes cultivating the positive in life. The wisdom and clarity that you uncover with the skill of awareness can be used to create what you want, from a positive relationship to food and your body to a greater sense of joy and delight in living. This is why mindfulness is also called "insight" practice. The more often you can be present without judgment, the more available you are to insights about how to guide your actions when you eat, move, and live in ways that reduce suffering and create greater happiness.

31. Choosing Happiness

Research has demonstrated that we are born with a set range of happiness—a range that is, thankfully, flexible. I'm not talking about the cheap-thrill version of happiness that you experience through the instant gratification of some desire—buying new clothes or shoes, eating a yummy piece of cake, having great sex, or winning at a board game. That type of happiness is based on a fleeting emotion that results from having a pleasant experience, like eating chocolate chip cookies fresh out of the oven. These moments of happiness are wonderful. In fact, the joyful moments with food are some of my biggest pleasures in daily life. But true happiness is not a food group.

The happiness I'm proposing is based on a decision and an approach to living that remains consistent through all of life's ups and downs. Pleasant *and* unpleasant experiences will always be a part of your everyday life, but happiness can steadily flow underneath the constant flux of ups and downs. Although achieving that might sound a little daunting, the really good news is that you don't have to wait on someone or something else to give it to you. You can live at the top of your happiness range through your own simple efforts and regardless of the situation.

I guess the first thing to consider is this: is happiness something you truly value? I have never talked to anyone who has said they would rather be unhappy than happy. But, sadly, the actions and thoughts of many people often reflect the opposite of what they really want. I think one reason for this disconnect between values life without letting them completely overwhelm you or habitually seeking comfort in trips to the kitchen. As you feel and let go of difficult emotions, you can cultivate whatever helps you thrive—creating balance as you ride the waves of life and make it to the shore without breaking your neck or your heart.

Setting the intention to be happy, because you have consciously decided happiness is something you value, is at the foundation of your psychological health and well-being as well as your ability to seek and find pleasure in a wide variety of ways. Here is your opportunity to set the course for your entire life. Do you have the courage and commitment to choose happiness? Choosing happiness can support your efforts to eat for pleasure and nourishment, live in your body with love, and color your life with gratitude and contentment.

Savoring Practice

First of all, set your general intention. This could sound something like "I commit to creating happiness by my response to life as it unfolds from moment to moment" or something as simple as "I choose to be happy." Take a moment and write down in your own words the intention you wish to make. Place the piece of paper by your computer, on your nightstand, on the refrigerator, or somewhere else where you can see it and read it daily. Consciously connect to this value and notice how it begins to permeate your day, gladden your heart, and even help you pause before reaching for food to see whether this is the choice that will bring happiness.

32.　The Power of a Smile

One of my favorite mindfulness practices is smiling. I suggest that people smile while they hold a yoga pose, in stress reduction classes to counteract anxiety, and in mindful eating classes to transform difficult emotions and bring joy to the dinner table. And, to my amazement, there are people who actually resist doing it. Suggesting that you bring a smile to your face, as simple as turning up the two corners of your mouth, can be a little challenging and frightening to folks who aren't accustomed to such a practice.

To be fair, there is some indication that smiling in order to cover up underlying anger or resentment isn't all that helpful, particularly if you are really faking it and don't have any intention to be happy. But the larger body of evidence confirms a strong mind-body connection between the mere act of smiling and feeling better as a result. For instance, smiling triggers the release of endorphins, dopamine, and serotonin—hormones known to be essential in the regulation of positive emotions and motivation. These are powerful party animals waiting to help you feel better!

You don't even have to *feel* happy when you start to smile. Any type of deliberate smile can turn down the stress and anxiety and turn up the loving feelings. Shifting your face into a smiling position—I call it smile yoga—will activate the same regions in the brain as a spontaneous smile resulting from a pleasant experience. Your brain does not distinguish between a voluntary and an involuntary smile, and you will feel better.

intervention group, who practiced a five-minute smiling meditation three times per day over a period of seven consecutive days, experienced significantly increased mindfulness, gratitude, and compassion for others compared to a control group. Mindfulness was the key to increasing the benefits of smiling, through the awareness and savoring of pleasant sensations and accompanying thoughts and emotions.

As Thích Nhät Hanh says "Sometimes your joy is the source of your smile, but sometimes your smile can be the source of your joy." This simple, natural way of improving how you feel can boost your mood without food, caffeine, shopping, Facebooking, or any other quick-fix strategies that have less staying power.

Savoring Practice

You can practice smiling any time, any place, but here's a smile meditation adapted from Pamela's study that you can do before you eat. It takes only a minute to change the whole experience of dining.

At mealtime, sit down in a comfortable position at the table. Close your eyes and take a moment to connect with yourself as you are right now. Bring your attention to your breath and take a couple of deep inhales and full exhales. Now gently let go of the awareness of your breath, and very slowly bring a soft smile to your lips. Allow your smile to gradually grow bigger. Notice what happens in your face, in your heart, and in the rest of your body. Allow this smiling state to spread throughout your entire body, from head to toe. Infuse your heart, your

33. Just for Me!

When you do something creative, positive, uplifting, enjoyable, and fun, you are building up what I call your *emotional bank account.* These "just for me!" activities (as I call them) help you create and maintain emotions that boost your emotional "money in the bank." You do them for yourself and by yourself, cultivating the most important of all relationships—the one with yourself. Building up an emotional buffer of positive feelings makes it less likely that you will succumb to handy snacks or the takeout window when faced with difficult emotions.

This concept is discussed in a book by Jim Loehr and Tony Schwartz, *The Power of Full Engagement: Managing Energy, Not Time, Is the Key to High Performance and Personal Renewal.* They describe four kinds of energy that need to be renewed on a regular basis: physical, emotional, mental, and spiritual. They explain that "from an energy perspective, negative emotions are costly and inefficient." Conversely, your emotional energy is buoyed by activities that are pleasurable, renewing, and nourishing.

When you build up your emotional bank account with positive thoughts and experiences, this improves your psychological wellness set point and creates stronger resilience. When this baseline of wellness is higher, challenging situations will affect you, but you will be able to bounce back more effectively and quickly. This ability to more quickly recover from stress is often seen in people who meditate, exercise, and engage in activities that nourish them.

eat differently and explore new cuisines, but making choices based on your own taste buds can be a powerful step toward claiming your right to be curious and to please your body.

If you're still saying "Oh, I don't have time for that," you need to do this more than anyone. Taking time to go for a walk, cook a meal that pleases you, or other actions that bring you joy is one of the most important things that you can do for your well-being, and ultimately it will improve your ability to get all of those pressing things done, once you get back to them. Busy people require "just for me" time to stay sane and successful....

...And right at that point, I stopped pushing forward with my writing and went out for a walk by myself to soak up the sunshine. During that time, I came up with an idea for an article, heard some inspiring messages on a podcast from one of my favorite meditation teachers, and became more energized and relaxed for the rest of my day. I now feel in less of a hurry. I feel gratitude for the time I spent with myself, and I didn't turn to food to help me feel energized or avoid working.

What have you done for yourself today—just for you?

It is quite surprising to me that, when I ask people in my classes if they regularly engage in activities that are enjoyable and enriching, they often look confused. Their confusion is a sad commentary on how disconnected they have become from their source of joy. So I ask them to make a weekly practice of "just for me" activities and see what happens. They often come back beaming with delight at rediscovering an old family recipe or reclaiming a lost activity, or from the courage it took to try something new.

34. Strike a Yoga Pose, Do a Dance

Constantly struggling with your body by *telling* it your negative opinions or disappointments with it blocks your ability to hear the constant information download you *receive* from your body. A great way to reduce the negative self-talk is to stop, listen, and be guided by your body's wisdom through practices of embodied movement, like yoga, dance, tai chi, and qigong.

The very definition of yoga from Patanjali's yoga sutras is "the cessation of the fluctuations of the mind." That blew me away when I first heard it. This means that when you stop paying attention to and identifying with all the passing thoughts in your mind (which are often negative), there is a sense of peace, stillness, and happiness. And the method for taking your attention away from the thoughts is to take your attention to something else—namely your breath and body sensations.

There are many ways of becoming more in touch with your body, but doing it in a way that includes movement is particularly effective in increasing your physical and psychological well-being. For instance, one study investigated three common meditation practices (sitting meditation, body scan, and mindful yoga) to see if they produced different outcomes. After three weekly one-hour sessions, all practices were associated with a reduction in obsessive thinking and increases in self-compassion and psychological well-being. However, mindful yoga produced significantly greater increases in psychological well-being than did the other two practices.

1. Sit in an upright, but comfortable position on a chair or on a cushion on the floor—lengthen your spine and reach the crown of the head upward.

2. Bring your attention to your breath, and slowly and gently begin to deepen the inhale and the exhale. On the inhale, expand your belly, then your ribs, then your upper chest. Exhale from your upper chest, then your ribs, and then your belly—pulling your belly button toward your spine to release all of the air from your body. Repeat a few times until you feel calmer and more grounded.

3. Take a deep breath in as you stretch your arms out to the side and overhead. Exhale as you bring your arms back to your sides. Coordinate the movement of your arms with your breath and repeat five times.

4. Bring your right arm overhead and your left hand to your side as you lean to the left for a stretch along the right side of your body. Hold and breathe for three long, steady breaths. Repeat on the other side.

5. Move your right ear over your right shoulder and make tiny circles with your chin. Be gentle with yourself. The neck is a very tender location for most of us. Repeat on the other side as you continue to take long, steady breaths.

6. Roll your shoulders backward in a circle nine times as you continue to breathe deeply.

I can be found doing yoga poses standing in line at the grocery store and dancing my way through life with music over the intercom in many offices and stores. Dare to break out of your shell, get creative, and discover the joy of moving.

long it takes for neural networks to begin to rewire themselves in the body" and an attitude of gratitude to be established.

Gratitude can also change your view of your body. One study had participants come up with at least five things that they were grateful for in their bodies (such as the health, physical appearance, or functionality of their bodies) and take a minute to picture them in their minds. After that, they chose at least three of them and wrote why they were grateful for those things. As a result, participants reported significantly greater satisfaction with their weight, significantly more favorable evaluation of their appearance, and greater body satisfaction compared to participants in the control condition. Another study, which compared gratitude to a cognitive restructuring therapy, found gratitude more effective at increasing body esteem, decreasing body dissatisfaction, reducing dysfunctional eating, and reducing depressive symptoms.

Mealtime is a great time to practice reflecting on gratitude. At your next meal, before you start to eat, take stock of how grateful you are for this food. Take a moment to be grateful for each step in the food process—for the seeds and the soil they were planted in, the rain that helped the seeds to grow, the sun and the weather that was needed for the plants to flourish, the farmers who grew and harvested the food, the truck driver who drove the produce to the store, the clerks at the grocery store who stocked the shelves, the store clerk who checked you out, and the person (maybe you) who prepared the food. Be aware of your interconnectedness with the world around you through the food you eat, and give thanks for the nourishment you are about to receive.

you want, you are acting as if you have already received it, and this energy of receiving puts you in the perfect place to reap results. And, let's face it, no matter whether you get exactly what you thought you wanted, you are happier anyway because the attitude of gratitude—and saying "thanks"—is, in itself, a balm that heals.

you meet my conditions and love me back in a certain way" or "You'll be worthy of my love when you can fit into those pants from five years ago." It's not romantic love, where you have an attraction for a specific someone, idealizing them for the time that the fascination is aroused. In other words, it's not love that is needy, attached, conditional, selfish, or dependent on conditions.

Loving-kindness is mindfulness with an emphasis on the heart. The heart's kindness and compassion sometimes takes second place during the modern practice of mindfulness, which emphasizes the aspect of being present. However, Dipa Ma, a famous meditation teacher from India, said, "From my own experience, there is no difference between mindfulness and loving kindness." Amita Schmidt, an American meditation teacher who wrote a book about her, said, "For [Dipa Ma], love and awareness were one. When you are fully loving, aren't you also mindful? When you are mindful, is this not also the essence of love?"

The repetition of phrases of loving-kindness is used in the practice so that you can strengthen your focus and concentration. The phrases are not set in stone, but there are similarities from teacher to teacher, person to person. I have developed my version of the phrases that resonate most with me, and I'll share them with you here. Of course, feel free to change the wording as you like.

May you be safe and protected, from inner and outer harm.

May you be peaceful and content, with things as they are.

May you be healthy and strong, as you are capable of being.

called Body Loving-Kindness that goes along with this chapter, at http://www.LynnRossy.com/multimedia, or you can read these instructions and practice on your own.

Close your eyes and bring your attention to your heart center. Take a deep breath in and then let it go with a sigh. Bring to mind a time when you felt unconditionally loved by someone—an aunt or uncle, grandma or grandpa, mom or dad, or your favorite pet. Intensify the feelings of being loved by remembering times you had together, when you were held with unreserved and unqualified care and attention. You might even gently rest your hands over your heart. Feel your chest expanding on the inbreath and deflating on the outbreath.

As you continue to breathe, softly offer the following phrases to yourself. Imagine them being offered into your heart.

May I be safe and protected.

May I be peaceful and content.

May I be healthy and strong.

May I live with joy and ease.

Repeat them over and over to yourself. Take your time. There is no hurry.

Pause at the end of each phrase and imagine the wishes moving into your body, through your heart, and infusing every cell with goodness and light—from head to toe to fingertip. Continue for as long as you wish. Then move into your day surrounded by loving energy.

when it was happening. This reflection of yourself as skillful, successful, adept, caring, sensitive, trustworthy, and so on can help you form a more rounded perspective on yourself. Reflecting and cultivating this sense of your worth is truly necessary, since your mind (like all minds) will latch onto the negative and slide right past the positive.

Think about all of the times you've beaten yourself up for overeating or eating "bad" food. I'm going to guess that this has happened before! Now turn it around. Start with acknowledging one instance when you spent the appropriate time to check in with your body about what it wanted to eat, fed yourself accordingly, and stopped before you were too full. Reflect on how it felt to be in this friendly connection with your body. Reflect on the food that you ate and how you felt afterward. The more vividly you can relive the experience, the easier it will be for you to recreate it. How would you feel if you did that more often?

Acknowledge all of the other ways that you have taken care of your body—times when you took your body out for a walk, when you bought your body some new clothes that you felt good in, and when you took care of your body by giving yourself enough rest. Can you remember looking in the mirror and saying, "Hey there! I really like you"? What did your body feel like, what emotions were present, and what were you thinking? Acknowledging yourself and the things you do every day to support your well-being can begin to build on itself. If it feels good and you take time to acknowledge it, you are more likely to repeat it.

38. Assume Authority. Act Until Apprehended

At the wellness program where I worked, we were going through a tumultuous time. In just a year, we had gone through four different managers who didn't know all that much about leading a wellness team. Each week during our team meetings that weren't attended by the "boss," it was clear that everyone was confused, conflicted, and unsure about how to proceed on a number of projects. In the past, we would have relied on our original director, who was highly intelligent and effective at her job. But she was long gone. What to do?

Out of my mouth came "Assume authority. Act until apprehended." Everyone paused with their mouths hanging open for a second, and then smiles began to creep onto their faces.

"Yes!" they shouted, "That's what we should do."

I basically just gave them permission to do what they already knew how to do but weren't trusting themselves to do. It was a game changer for our team. We became productive and efficient again.

Jennifer, who was a part of the wellness team that day, said this about it: "These are powerful words. I truly believe this to be a life-changing philosophy for me personally and empowering to women, who often wait for permission to just be a human being. I no longer feel the need for that level of validation. I repeat those words— 'Assume authority, act until apprehended'—frequently to this day! And, yes, I am rarely apprehended!"

How could it be that you should be someone different from who you are? It's impossible. Embrace the beauty of every part of your body—size, age, hair, wrinkles, color. Each human being is a breath of the divine, and as long as you're breathing, your sacred duty is to care for and love yourself. This requires that you assume authority for your body and how it looks, and treat it with honor and kindness.

Now, I want to warn you. Once you start assuming authority for how you eat and your body, your whole life might start to change. In fact, as you take this motto into other areas of your life, all hell may break loose (in a good way!). When you act without seeking other people's approval or authority, you might be pleasantly surprised at the results. What do you really want to do? I often like to ask people: "What would you do if you weren't afraid?" Be brave, and act until apprehended.

Savoring Practice

The next time you catch yourself looking for someone else's opinion about aspects of how you should eat or look, stop and pause. Repeat the words *Assume authority. Act until apprehended.* Put aside everything that you've heard, and take a moment to tap into your body's wisdom and your heart's intuition. What is it telling you? How is it guiding you? You might notice fear or confusion at first, telling you it's not safe to act in this way. Acknowledge the feelings and then let them go. Stop and pause again. Take a deep breath. Ask again. Keep asking until you feel a sense of calm arising from within. When you are in deep

39. Cultivate Contentment

After many years of practicing meditation, I discovered the beauty of contentment. I think it took me so long to notice because contentment is not flashy or bold. It doesn't call out for your attention, like when you're experiencing something really pleasant or unpleasant. No, the experience of being contented requires that you make a little effort to acknowledge and cultivate it. That's why I consider the practice of cultivating contentment to be an advanced mindfulness practice and one of the most profound and healing ones I've learned.

At a retreat led by Christina Feldman, I was given meditation instructions that focused on being aware of pleasant sensations, unpleasant sensations, and neutral (neither pleasant or unpleasant) sensations. We were to pay attention to each experience and then notice the effect that followed. As I mentioned in chapter 13, pleasant sensations often lead to "wanting more" (or craving), unpleasant sensations often lead to "wanting less" (or pushing away), and neutral sensations often lead to "delusion" (or boredom, confusion). However, what I discovered that day, as I dropped deeply into the neutral moments, was not confusion or boredom, but a profound sense of contentment. When I shared my insight to the group after the meditation, Christina simply said "Yes, dear. That's what I notice too."

You can use any moment in life to cultivate contentment. First of all, let's examine the pleasant experiences in life. For example, grabbed by something pleasant or resisting something unpleasant. These are the moments when you're making the bed, making coffee, taking a shower, walking from place to place, driving in the car, washing the dishes, sweeping the floor, turning on your computer, reading your email, getting dressed, washing the clothes, doing the grocery shopping, picking up the kids from school, and on and on.

You can make all of these moments into something pleasant or unpleasant by the thoughts and stories in your head. But if you can catch yourself and be present with what's happening without the story line, there is nothing to grasp at and nothing to push away. Contentment is this sense of well-being that comes from knowing that this moment doesn't need to be any different from how it is. Pleasant and unpleasant feelings can come and go, and you're not reacting. And when things are more neutral, you don't "fall asleep" by getting lost in your head. Pay attention to what you're doing, and immerse yourself in the present moment with relaxed attention. Over time, boredom becomes contentment, which begins to be shaded around the edges with pleasantness.

Savoring Practice

Spend some time noticing moments of contentment that are already available to you. These are especially present in the ordinary moments of your day. Instead of labeling these as dull or boring, sense the preciousness of moments not colored by the stronger energies of pleasant and unpleasant. Then spend some time cultivating contentment.

40. The Keys to Happiness

In mindfulness-based communities, there is a well-known teaching called *the keys to happiness.* I have used them to help me run a mindfulness center, direct my career, be in relationships, and even eat. They were developed by Angeles Arrien, a cultural anthropologist, award-winning author, and educator who originally called them the four-fold way: (1) show up and choose to be present, (2) pay attention to what has heart and meaning, (3) tell your truth without blame or judgment, and (4) be open to outcome, not attached to outcome.

I have already talked a lot about showing up for your life and choosing to be present. All good things come from this first key task. And while that might sound simplistic, as I've mentioned, we are not present about half of the time, and therefore we aren't practicing one of the most essential steps toward happiness. When you're only half present while eating, you're not tasting or enjoying nearly as much as you could. You may not be paying attention to the signals from your belly that indicate it's had enough. Or you may be ignoring signs that the food doesn't really taste good. For eating to be an opportunity for nourishment and pleasure, every aspect of the eating experience requires your attention. Otherwise it quickly devolves into a mindless act with dubious consequences.

Paying attention to what has heart and meaning helps you to direct your activities and decisions based on what adds value to your life and away from the ones that are less important. In general, you can apply this teaching to help you stop at any moment and future you can't even imagine. Saying no limits you to what you've done before. Do the same thing and get the same results. But when you show up, pay attention, tell your truth, and become open to the outcome, your boat will be following the current of opportunity as you ride along the river of life.

Savoring Practice

Before you eat, stop and pause. Consciously choose to be present for the experience of noticing your hunger, picking the food that you want to eat, preparing or buying the food, and preparing the place where you will eat so that it supports enjoyment and presence (for example, removing cellphones, books, and computers from the table).

How can you bring more heart and meaning into your mealtime? Perhaps you want to pause and say thanks before the meal. Or to eat something solely to nourish your body, or solely for pleasure, or both. Allow space for questions and answers to arise. Remember, you are being guided by *your* truth, not someone else's idea about what you should do. Can you claim your truth with food and relax into that knowing? Finally, be open to the outcome. Be open to the experience of eating. Each bite is a unique opportunity to savor and enjoy.

Other Savoring Practices: Use the keys to the four-fold way to happiness in the rest of your life and see how they alter and shift your experience of what it means to be fully engaged. Spend some time in reflection. What could you do to be more present? Meditate? Do yoga? What already has heart and meaning in your life, and what could you do to foster more of this in your life? What is *your* truth in each

Savor Every Moment

Be it tart or sweet, always savor the moment. You'll not taste one just like it again.

—Erica Alex

What does it mean, to savor? Here's a definition from positive psychology: "When one savors, one is aware of pleasure and appreciates the positive feelings one is experiencing." This implies that you could be *experiencing* something pleasant but not *savoring* it, because you aren't even aware of it, much less appreciating it. Thus the important ingredients for savoring are both your presence *and* your appreciation when pleasant sensations arise.

While we don't deny that there are challenging, difficult aspects of life, your attention to savoring can enhance your ability to see how often and under what circumstances the pleasures in life occur. Fleeting pleasures of tasty food, buying new shoes, or getting a raise (hedonic pleasures) as well as deeper pleasures resulting from meaningful work, generosity, and a value-driven life (eudaimonic pleasures) can both be experienced to produce an additive effect instead of sacrificing one for the other.

41. Savor Every Bite

Have you ever observed that food pops into your mouth before you know what's happened? Or have you suddenly become aware, during a meal, that you're starting to feel pretty full or maybe even a little sick from how much food you've eaten? Believe me, you're not alone. Even during my mindful eating presentations, in which conscious eating is the focus, I have watched people be unaware of eating.

I'll never forget the first time it happened. I was teaching the BASICS of Mindful Eating to participants in a workshop and had asked people to come to the front and choose a couple of pieces of chocolate to take back to their seats so that we could practice together. Sharon picked up a piece of chocolate and unconsciously threw it into her mouth while she was walking past me. I saw the chocolate as it was flying through the air from her hand to her mouth and said "Wait! We're going to eat together as a group." She looked a little embarrassed, but I laughed and told her to get another piece. After the exercise, Sharon exclaimed, "What a difference! I didn't taste the first one I popped into my mouth at all, but the second one was full of taste—from the bitterness of chocolate, the texture from the nuts, and the bursts of flavor from the salt. It was delicious!"

How many bites do we miss? Well, probably quite a few. I've noted that about half of the time we're not present unless we make a conscious effort to the contrary. Simple habituation to routine activities like eating can decrease our sensitivity to the pleasure that

that coat your tongue—each one with fifty to a hundred taste cells folded together like the petals of a young flower about to bloom. These taste buds offer us the bitter, sweet, sour, salt, and umami (described as savory or "meaty") flavors we then savor. Knowing the details of this intricate process makes it even more extraordinary that you could possibly ignore the explosions of flavor that happen every time you put food into your mouth.

A final way of having pleasure can be remembering past moments of savoring food. You can remember a great meal at a favorite restaurant, a comfort meal cooked by your mother, or a special treat that you had when you were on vacation. For me, travel is mainly an opportunity to try delicious food from different cultures and regions of the country. Extend your ability to savor every bite by reminiscing about the pleasant food experiences you've already had.

Although you probably won't ever savor absolutely every bite, you can certainly increase the moments of savoring by paying more attention and appreciating the experience. As in every mindfulness exercise, it's important to notice when you're not paying attention and kindly and compassionately bring yourself back to the act of eating and appreciating, over and over again.

Savoring Practice

Here are some tips for enhancing your ability to savor every bite.

1. What can you do to improve the beauty of the environment where you eat? Putting a tablecloth down, setting the table

42. Savor the Food You Really Want

Do you find yourself eating the same food over and over again? You have the same food for breakfast, the same food for lunch, and sometimes mix it up a little at dinner. When you eat this way, it's no wonder you get a little bored and find it hard to pay attention. The ability to be present and appreciate what you're eating (the definition of savoring) requires that you put a little effort into the experience. Even if the food is pleasurable, if you repeat it too often you will habituate to it and find it harder to savor.

One way you can start to improve your practice of savoring every bite is to eat the food you really want. This means that instead of trying to eat "right," "good," "clean," or the way some diet tells you to eat, you are checking inside to see what really sounds good. You can savor the food that you really want much more easily than the food you think you have to have. And when you give yourself the food you really want, you are less likely to overeat, because you will be satisfied. No amount of rice cakes will satisfy your desire for chocolate if chocolate is what you want! So have the chocolate, or whatever else it is your body is really asking for.

The next question might be: "How do I do that?" Particularly if you haven't been listening to your body for how to eat, tapping into your body's wisdom will require that you take a journey down the road of many flavors. This is a beautiful travel requirement for

- Spices like cardamom, chiles, cilantro, cinnamon, cloves, coriander, cumin, curry, garlic, ginger, mint, mustard seeds, nutmeg, red pepper flakes, saffron, sesame seeds, and turmeric

Latino

- Cuban black beans, tamales, and enchiladas
- Spices like chiles, cilantro, cinnamon, cumin, garlic, oregano, and sesame seeds

Mediterranean

- Spanakopita, pizza, or lentil and vegetable stew
- Spices like basil, bay leaves, fennel, garlic, marjoram, mint, nutmeg, oregano, parsley, red pepper flakes, rosemary, saffron, sage, and thyme

Middle Eastern

- Hummus or baba ghanoush with pita, falafel, and gyros
- Spices like allspice, cilantro, cinnamon, coriander, cumin, garlic, marjoram, mint, oregano, sesame seeds, and thyme

Moroccan

- Lamb stew with couscous and meat or vegetable tagine
- Spices like cilantro, cinnamon, coriander, cumin, garlic, ginger, mint, red pepper flakes, saffron, thyme, and turmeric

If you have been depriving yourself of certain foods for a while (such as those with sugar and fat), you might find yourself craving them. Deprivation sets up craving and wanting. When you first allow yourself previously forbidden foods, it can feel overwhelming. Let yourself have what you want, but do so with mindfulness, kindness, and compassion, as best you can. Set up some structure around the eating experience so you have a reasonable serving. However, if you overdo a little, it won't kill you. And you are teaching yourself that you can have whatever you want, thus reducing the craving. Gradually you will notice that a wider variety of food becomes attractive and desirable.

- Are you feeling curious, fascinated, intrigued, involved, stimulated, or alert?

- Are you feeling proud, safe, or secure?

- Are you feeling amazed, aroused, astonished, dazzled, energetic, giddy, surprised, or passionate?

- Are you feeling appreciative, thankful, awed, or amazed?

- Are you feeling calm, content, mellow, satisfied, or serene?

- Are you feeling ecstatic, elated, radiant, or thrilled?

When you experience something pleasant, try to home in on the exact description of how you're feeling. You might need more than one feeling word to capture the entirety of your experience. Take your time to explore different words until you get it right. You might be feeling something because of what you've done, what someone else did, or what is happening in the environment. Open yourself up to being more attentive to when pleasant moments occur, and then give a juicy, descriptive name to how you're feeling.

By the way, women tend to be more adept at savoring than men, simply because—as studies show—they are more consciously aware of their feelings and share their feelings with others more often. This means that men will have to work a little harder. You can do it! I promise. All it takes is your willingness to try and your desire to be a little happier.

notice whether reliving the experience stimulates the pleasant feelings to arise again. By noticing and naming the feelings when you're having them *and* sharing them afterward with someone else, you double your pleasure and double your fun.

usual spunky self. And she said two things that have always stuck with me. First, she talked about how people like to complain about the weather, but now she realized "any weather is good weather." And second, she reflected on how she used to complain about her hair, but now "any hair is good hair." Those statements really put things into poignant perspective for me. In Buddhism, death is seen as one of our teachers, and Ginnie was showing me this in person.

The five reflections (from the Buddhist teachings) include knowing that we will die, knowing that we are subject to old age, knowing that we are not exempt from illness, knowing that we will be parted from those we love and things we love, and knowing that we are subject to the effects of our actions and behaviors. Knowing deeply the transitory nature of everything helps us to let go of needing things to be other than how they are and brings about a sense of lightness in our heart and minds. We are then in the state of mind to savor what is here in every moment—the good, the bad, and the ugly—without being in the grip of fear or hope. This is it! This is the way it is for everyone.

While that might sound a little depressing, it really isn't meant to be at all. In fact, once you stop denying the truth of death, aging, illness, impermanence, and the effect of your actions by examining them for yourself, you realize that you've just been given an amazing gift—the present moment and all that it has to offer. The wonderful moments are more precious, the difficult moments are forgiven, the neutral moments become grander by sensing into the contentment that they offer. In other words, they can each be savored as a part of the fabric of human life.

Your resistance might be about some aspect of your body, a moment of eating mindlessly, a conflict with a loved one or coworker, or a thousand other things you might resist about life. Let the resistance be your bell of mindfulness. Take a deep breath in and exhale fully. Do that as many times as you need, to sense some release.

Jon Kabat-Zinn wrote "As long as you are breathing, there is more right with you than wrong with you." As the breath relaxes you, remember the preciousness of your body just as it is; that eating mindlessly is normal, there is nothing wrong with conflict, and life can just be difficult sometimes. Remember, there is *always* a way of gaining a wider perspective on any situation.

as physically active, according to the Office of the Surgeon General. One group of housekeepers was not given this information. After just four weeks, the women who were taught to look at their activity differently experienced significant changes—losing an average of two pounds, lowering their blood pressure by almost 10 percent, and showing improvements in body-fat percentage, body mass index, and waist-to-hip ratio—compared to the control group. The interesting aspect of the study is that the housekeepers did not report any change in their activity, but they were taught to think differently about the activity they already did—having a new understanding that it counted.

In my classes, I suggest that people start with one extra movement activity that they will do over the coming week. People get very creative and do things like go to the bathroom in the building next door, walk an extra lap around the block before they go in the front door, park farther away from the store, and walk the dog willingly instead of arguing with their partner about who has to do it. At my house, I've quit complaining about my husband's leaving the lights on everywhere, including down in the basement. Now I just see it as an opportunity to walk up and down the stairs.

Being mindful has been shown to be associated with the maintenance of higher activity levels, for a number of interesting reasons. First of all, mindfulness teaches us to use a beginner's mind. Instead of discounting that an activity might be enjoyable, we are willing to give it a try before we make a judgment. Second, mindful attention makes it less likely you will hurt yourself. This is particularly important in our "no pain, no gain" world, where people tend to overdo it at first if they aren't paying careful attention. Third, when you

In each movement, remember to be aware of the sensations that arise, and appreciate the fact that your body *can* move. Remember, every movement counts. Instead of complaining about the times when you have to move or are forced to park farther away from your destination, see these as opportunities to savor movement. Look for even more opportunities to move throughout your day, being sure to give yourself credit for the fact that you're moving. Perhaps share a movement activity with someone else and talk to them about your experiment with savoring movement. Sharing your positive feelings with others enhances the joy!

prepares itself for food. Looking at food along the buffet line, at the grocery store, or in the bakery case does the same thing.

Even if you're not looking at the food, walking by a bakery and smelling the freshly baked breads, cakes, and cookies is one of the most potent sensory experiences you can have. My mouth is watering just thinking about it. Or what about the aroma of popcorn at the movie theater, BBQ ribs at the outdoor food stand, apple pie fresh out of the oven, and onion and garlic sizzling in olive oil as you start to prepare your meal. The sense of both taste and smell is targeted by food companies because they know how powerfully these senses pull us toward food and eating, even when we're not hungry. It's even been reported they put odor into food packaging to try to get us to eat more of it!

Lastly, let's consider the sound that food makes. Sound, according to Charles Spence, gastrophysicist and Professor of Experimental Psychology at the University of Oxford, is the "forgotten flavor" and has often been overlooked in the overall multisensory experience of food and eating. Most people report being unaware of the impact of sound on how they perceive and respond to food and drink. But think of those food advertisements on TV with the crispy, crunchy, and crackly sounds accentuated to grab your attention. A growing body of research has documented that the sounds produced by food strongly influence the perceived pleasure.

Seeing, smelling, and hearing food all can enhance our ability to savor food when we're hungry. But what about when we're not hungry? Those same senses are at work when you're not hungry and may influence you to eat anyway. I learned this lesson with

47. Savor One Thing at a Time

Besides practicing mindfulness with your eating senses, let's explore how mindfulness can be applied to other things that you do. Despite what many people seem to believe and flaunt as a badge of productivity, multitasking is not something humans do well. It doesn't stop them from trying, though. How many times have you tried to be on the phone, type an email, and read an article at the same time? (I'm guilty!) How much did you learn from the phone call, how many mistakes did you make typing your email, and how much information did you glean from that article? Probably not much. In fact, multitasking ends up taking up *more* of our time, because we have to go back and redo everything again with our full attention.

The same thing happens when cooking or eating. Have you ever noticed that your lack of attention had an unexpected punch when you put a tablespoon of chili powder in the chili instead of a teaspoon? Oops! Or when you're eating, how many times have you finished a full plate of food and not noticed any of the flavor that you could have savored, much less registered the signs of fullness setting in? You can eat (or drink) the same food for years and not really taste it. Jane said "After just one week (in the Eat for Life class), my diet soda is too sweet."

Our distractions and multitasking also impact our relationships with others—our children, partners, friends, and colleagues. Our inability to be present and listen has created chasms between us that sometimes lead to the ending of relationships or, at the very least, straining them through our inattention and lack of affection.

you fully immerse yourself in one activity or task so that you can either (1) savor it more deeply when it is pleasurable or (2) navigate it more easily, even though there might be challenges. Particularly when things are challenging, mindfulness can improve your capacity to stay present without resorting to habits like avoiding or procrastinating.

Focusing and maintaining your attention on pleasant moments increases the release of dopamine in your brain and strengthens the experience in your long-term memory. The longer you can hold something in your awareness, the more stimulating it is to the brain and the stronger the connection you'll have in your memory. For example, you could pay particular attention to the rewarding and pleasurable aspects of sitting out on the patio eating hot blueberry crisp, fresh out of the oven, with ice cream melting on top. You could feel the heat of the sun on your face, the crisp air of the spring day, and the fragrance of the lilac and viburnum wafting on the breeze. Just reading this, couldn't you taste, feel, and smell all of it, even though you weren't really there?

Using mindfulness to maintain your attention on the details of challenging situations, projects, or problems can help you move through unavoidable circumstances with more ease. Focusing on the details in front of you instead of focusing on the larger picture or your idea of what might happen in the future (which is what often makes us anxious) allows you to face each moment one step at a time. For example, if you have a project at work that needs to be finished, instead of spending an inordinate amount of time snacking in the break room as a way of avoiding, you can focus on the separate steps you need to take to complete the project. Not only

48. Savor Nature

One way to improve our ability to focus, relax our hurried minds, and appreciate our lives is to spend time in nature. When I'm scattered, anxious, and irritable, there is hardly anything better than a walk on one of the trails in the nearby woods. With no concrete in sight and only trees rustling in the wind, my mind begins to clear, and I slip into the calm peace of the natural surroundings. While walking on a city street will have its benefits, going into nature will reduce both the amount of pollution you breathe and the level of distraction and noise that you have to filter out. The canopy of the forest or park, the grandeur of the mountains, and the soothing quality of the beach all have sounds and sights that help calm our overtaxed nervous systems.

Going into nature for the physical and psychological benefits it offers has been given a lot of attention, particularly by the Japanese government, which coined the term shinrin-yoku or "forest bathing" all the way back in 1982. As our modern lives continue to become more stressful (think of the pandemic that spread around the globe in 2020!), it increases in importance. A recent systematic review of medical research on forest bathing demonstrated many benefits, including significantly improved physical health markers and emotional states, physical and psychological recovery, and adaptive behaviors, as well as a reduction of anxiety and depression. I won't blame you if you set down the book right now and stroll off into the nearest forest!

will be enhanced through your time spent in nature. You will feel more grounded while standing steady on the earth and less likely to reach for food or other fleeting fixes when you're feeling down or stressed. You will be more flexible during the ebb and flow of your emotions and the changing winds of circumstance.

Savoring Practice

Pick a place in nature that feels safe to you. Fill up a water bottle, and if you must take your phone, turn it off or choose a setting without beeps or vibrations. Of course, when you're going into a park or forest, even if you've been there a number of times before, let someone know where you're going and when you'll return. You can take something inspiring to read or a journal to write in.

Okay, you're ready. Head out to your destination and leave behind any expectations or goals. Start walking, and let your body guide you in choosing which path to take. You can borrow the main principles used by forest bathers: to breathe, relax, wander, touch, listen, and heal. Take your time. This isn't a race. At some point your body will find a place that calls out to you to stop and rest. Pause to look more closely at the sky, the trees, the creeks, and the animals. Notice the smells of the trees, the flowers, and the air. Use all of your senses to take in the totality of the nature around you. Use this time to immerse yourself fully in the experience and appreciate the beauty of life all around you. Write or draw in your journal the impressions that you feel or see as you bathe your senses.

49. Savor Generosity

When you are feeling lonely or deprived, or like you don't have "enough," one of the best ways to fill yourself up is not with food (believe it or not!) but by looking outside of yourself, by engaging in acts of kindness and giving to others. Of course, we have all been told that generosity is a noble and moral act. For instance, it may be common for you to make meals for people who are sick or for those grieving a loss, give monetary support during an emergency crisis, give time or money to charities and nonprofits, or tithe at your place of worship.

The practice of "giving where you are spiritually fed" is found in Buddhism through the practice of dãna, the Pali word for generosity. Many Buddhist teachers live solely on dãna, in the form of monetary support from the students who receive their teachings, given at the end of each retreat, workshop, or talk. Each student is asked to look into his heart to explore what is the right amount for him to give in return for the most precious gift—the gift of the teachings. Can you imagine living on dãna? That would be like waiting on your boss to decide how much they feel moved to pay you at the end of each month. It's a truly humbling and awe-inspiring tradition that is carried on to this day.

The benefits of generosity came into clear focus for me as the forced isolation that began during the coronavirus pandemic lingered on and on. Being someone with a lot of privilege during this time (for example, my household had regular income, we had a farmer delivering food, my mortgage was paid), it felt

and the happiness that you gave the recipient. We all have gifts to give if we open our hearts and become willing to look beyond our self-interest or self-absorption and into the hearts and lives of others. When we fill ourselves by giving to others, the emptiness inside ourselves begins to disappear. Filling yourself through savoring your acts of generosity can be a gracious habit that replaces filling yourself with things you don't really need.

Savoring Practice

Take the generosity challenge of thirty days of giving. Start with the simple question of *Where can I give?* and be open to the miracles that happen as occasions to give offer themselves to you. It might be a fundraiser on Facebook for someone's birthday, a fundraising letter or text, or a chance to help someone in need. Don't hesitate to act when you hear of an opportunity to be generous. And if you feel a tightening or clenching related to the act of giving, ask yourself what would happen if you could be open instead. Do something—big or small—each day. Let yourself savor—be present to and appreciative of—each moment of the giving. Sense your connectedness to the other, to the community, and to the world. As you send your gifts, your receipt is already resting in your heart.

I took a picture of the gifts I gave for thirty days, and it made a wonderful collage of loving deeds. This act was not for a gratuitous pat on the back, but as a way of helping me acknowledge there was a vast world now living inside of my heart. Loneliness cannot enter where there is no empty room to fill.

your job and taking a trip around the world that you always wanted. (Although, maybe.) It's more likely, however, that through the recognition that you have only moments to live you might see more clearly the glimmers of light around the most important things you could be giving your attention.

Savoring life can also happen more deeply if you imagine, for instance, that this is the last time you will ever do a particular activity. Notice what kind of attention and curiosity arises when you bring that consideration to the table. A last cup of coffee, a last hike through the woods, the last full moon rising in the evening sky, the last conversation with a friend or touch from a loved one—all things become more exquisitely real and poignant when we come alive to our impermanence. This is meant not to depress you, but to increase your appreciation of and attention to the pleasure you might be completely missing.

If you really want to jump into the deep end of the pool, I suggest you attend a silent meditation or yoga retreat. In my experience, that is when the deepest insights and discoveries happen, the ones that are the most life changing. The length of time can vary from a day to much longer. Mine have mostly been of the seven to nine day variety. These periods of retreat offer fewer distractions, more spacious time, and a precious opportunity in which to examine yourself—teaching you so much more about mindfulness than what you'll read in a book. Of course, sitting and savoring your life with full attention and appreciation for a few moments each day might be enough to wake you up in unimaginable ways.

The peaceful stillness that you tap into when you come home to yourself helps you to discover the friend you've been as you settle fully into your body and into the present moment.

Relax. Breathing deeply will automatically help you feel relaxed, but let's bring that relaxation into the nooks and crannies of your body. Invite it in. Bring a sense of relaxation into the muscles of your face; neck and shoulders; chest and belly; arms, hands, and fingers; legs, feet, and toes. Let them all soften and relax. Pay particular attention to any tension you might be holding in your jaw, neck, shoulders, and belly. Keep breathing, softening, and relaxing.

Feel. Welcome any emotions that are present as if they were guests of honor. Welcome everything and reject nothing for the full experience of being alive. How does it feel to open in this way? What is the quality of your heart? Is it open, closed, tight, or neutral? Simply breathe, relax, and feel whatever arises and allow it to be held in the gentle embrace of your attention.

Watch. Watch the passing show of body sensations, thoughts, and emotions. The witnessing part of you is completely without judgment and full of love and compassion for all that you are, watching all that arises, exists, and passes away, from moment to moment. Experience both the pleasure and the pain more fully from this place of greater acceptance and watchfulness. Watching doesn't mean you are disconnected from your life, but you are able to have a wider perspective when you stand back a little and watch the passing show.

Acknowledgments

To my dear partner, Bud, who wakes up happy every day and teaches me the true miracle of love. To my mom and dad, for teaching love by example. To twelve-step programs, for saving my life. To my Buddhist teachers, for guiding me on the path to end suffering. To my Kripalu yoga teachers, who taught me meditation in motion and guided me to the love and joy within. To the board of the Center for Mindful Eating, for being stewards of the practices that end suffering around food and the body.

References

Step One

Andre, C. 2011. *Looking at Mindfulness: 25 Ways to Live in the Moment Through Art.* New York: Blue Rider Press, 132.

Asurion. "Americans Don't Want to Unplug from Phones While on Vacation, Despite Latest Digital Detox Trend." May 17, 2018.

Deloitte Development LLC. 2018. 2018 Global Mobile Consumer Survey, US edition. https://www2.deloitte.com/tr/en/pages/technology-media-and-telecommunications/articles/global-mobile-consumer-survey-us-edition.html.

Fredrickson, B. L. 2017. "Your Phone vs. Your Heart." In *Future Directions in Well-Being,* edited by M. White, G. Slemp, and A. Murray. New York, NY: Springer.

Gallup Organization. 2019. Gallup Global Emotions Report. Washington, DC: Gallup Organization.

Killingsworth, M. A., and D. T. Gilbert. 2010. "A Wandering Mind Is an Unhappy Mind." *Science* 330(6006), 932.

Ma, X., Z. Yue, and Z. Gong. 2017. "The Effect of Diaphragmatic Breathing on Attention, Negative Affect, and Stress in Healthy Adults." *Frontiers in Psychology* 8, 874.

Roberts, J. A., and M. E. David, 2016. "My Life Has Become a Major Distraction from My Cell Phone: Partner Phubbing and Relationship Satisfaction Among Romantic Partners." *Computers in Human Behavior* 54, 134–141.

Scott, K. A., S. J. Melhorn, and R. R. Sakai. 2012. "Effects of Chronic Social Stress on Obesity." *Current Obesity Reports* 1(1) (March), 16–25.

Statista. 2020. Number of mobile phone users in the U.S. from 2012 to 2020. https://www.statista.com/statistics/222306/forecast-of-smartphone-users-in-the-us/.

Uvnäs-Moberg, K.,. L. Handlin, and M. Petersson. 2015. "Self-soothing Behaviors with Particular Reference to Oxytocin Release Induced by Non-noxious Sensory Stimulation." *Frontiers in Psychology* 5, 1529.

Step Three

Brennan, M. A., W. Icon, W. J. Whelton, and D. Sharpe. 2020. "Benefits of Yoga in the Treatment of Eating Disorders: Results of a Randomized Controlled Trial." *Eating Disorders.* https://doi:10.108 0/17439760.2019.1651888, doi:10.1080/10640266.2020.1731921.

Bucchianeri, M. M., and D. Newmark-Sztainer. 2014. Body Dissatisfaction: An Overlooked Public Health Concern." *Journal of Public Mental Health* 13, 64–69.

Butryn, M. L., A. Juarascio, J. Shaw, S. G. Kerrigan, V. Clark, O. O'Planick, and E. M. Forman. 2013. "Mindfulness and Its Relationship with Eating Disorders Symptomatology in Women Receiving Residential Treatment." *Eating Behaviors* 14, 13–16.

Oldham-Cooper, R. E., C. A. Hardman, C. E. Nicoll, P. J. Rogers, and J. M. Brunstrom. 2011. "Playing a Computer Game During Lunch Affects Fullness, Memory for Lunch, and Later Snack Intake." *American Journal of Clinical Nutrition,* 93(2), 308–313.

Richo, D. 2002. *How to Be an Adult in Relationships: The Five Keys to Mindful Loving.* Boston, MA: Shambala.

Rossy, L. 2016. *The Mindfulness-Based Eating Solution: Proven Strategies to End Overeating, Satisfy Your Hunger, and Savor Your Life.* Oakland, CA: New Harbinger.

Swami, V., L. Weis, D. Barron, and A. Furnham. 2018. "Positive Body Image Is Positively Associated with Hedonic (Emotional) and Eudemonic (Psychological and Social) Well-being in British Adults." *Journal of Social Psychology* 158(5), 541–552.

Tylka, T. L., and K. J. Homan. 2015. "Exercise Motives and Positive Body Image in Physically Active College Women and Men: Exploring an Expanded Acceptance Model of Intuitive Eating." *Body Image* 15, 90–97.

Lane, R. D. 2000. "Neural Correlates of Conscious Emotional Experience." In *Cognitive Neuroscience of Emotion*, edited by R. D. Lane and L. Nadel (pp. 345–370). New York: Oxford University Press.

Little, A. C., B. D. Jones, and L. M. DeBruine. 2011. "Facial Attractiveness: Evolutionary Based Research." *Philosophical Transaction of the Royal Society* 366: 1638–1659.

Loehr, J., and T. Schwartz. 2003. *The Power of Full Engagement: Managing Energy, Not Time, Is the Key to High Performance and Personal Renewal.* New York, NY: The Free Press.

Lyubomirsky, S., K. M. Sheldon, and D. Schkade. 2005. "Pursuing Happiness: The Architecture of Sustainable Change." *Review of General Psychology* 9(2). https://doi.org/10.1037/1089-2680.9.2.111.

Nettle, D. 2006. *Happiness: The Science Behind Your Smile.* Oxford: Oxford University Press.

Sauer-Zavala, S. E., E. C. Walsh, T. A. Eisenlohr-Moul, and E.L.B. Lykins. 2013. "Comparing Mindfulness-Based Intervention Strategies: Differential Effects of Sitting Meditation, Body Scan, and Mindful Yoga." *Mindfulness* 4, 383–388.

Schmidt, A. 2005. *Dipa Ma: The Life and Legacy of a Buddhist Master.* Cambridge: Windhorse Publications.

Strasser, P. 2017. "Meditative Smiling—A Path to Wellbeing." MAPP, University of East London, School of Psychology. https://www.makelifegr8.com/wp-content/uploads/2018/10/Research-Embodied-Positive-Mindfulness.pdf.

Wolfe, W. L., and K. Patterson. 2017. Comparison of a Gratitude-based and Cognitive Restructuring Intervention for Body Dissatisfaction and Dysfunctional Eating Behavior in College Women. *Eating Disorders* 25(4), 330–344. https://doi:10.1080/10640266.2017.1279908.

Spence, C. 2015. "Eating with Our Ears: Assessing the Importance of the Sounds of Consumption on Our Perception and Enjoyment of Multisensory Flavour Experiences." *Flavour* 4, 3. https://doi.org /10.1186/2044-7248-4-3.

Ulmer, C. S., B. A. Stetson, and P. G. Salmon, 2010. "Mindfulness and Acceptance Are Associated with Exercise Maintenance in YMCA Exercisers." *Behaviour Research and Therapy* 48(8), 805–809. https:// doi.org/10.1016/j.brat.2010.04.009.

Villablanca, P. A., et al. 2015. "Nonexercise Activity Thermogenesis in Obesity Management." *Mayo Clinic Proceedings* 90(4), 509–519.

Wen, Y., Q. Yan, Y. Pan, X. Gu, and Y. Liu. 2019. "Medical Empirical Research on Forest Bathing (Shinrin-yoku): A Systematic Review." *Environmental Health and Preventive Medicine* 24, 70. https://doi.org/10 .1186/s12199-019-0822-8.

Lynn Rossy, PhD, is a licensed clinical psychologist and author of *The Mindfulness-Based Eating Solution*. She developed Eat for Life, a research-based mindful eating program that helps you end over-eating, appreciate your body, and savor your life. She is president of The Center for Mindful Eating.